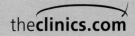
theclinics.com

RADIOLOGIC CLINICS
OF NORTH AMERICA

Neuroradiology Essentials

Guest Editor
RONALD L. WOLF, MD, PhD

January 2006 • Volume 44 • Number 1

IA# CRAD 3383387-101

CME

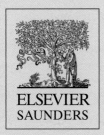
ELSEVIER
SAUNDERS

An imprint of Elsevier, Inc
PHILADELPHIA LONDON TORONTO MONTREAL SYDNEY TOKYO

W.B. SAUNDERS COMPANY
A Division of Elsevier Inc.

1600 John F. Kennedy Boulevard • Suite 1800 • Philadelphia, Pennsylvania 19103-2899

http://www.theclinics.com

RADIOLOGIC CLINICS OF NORTH AMERICA Volume 44, Number 1
January 2006 ISSN 0033-8389, ISBN 1-4160-3384-X

Editor: Barton Dudlick

Radiologic Clinics of North America (ISSN 0033-8389) is published bimonthly by W.B. Saunders Company. Corporate and editorial offices: 1600 John F. Kennedy Boulevard, Suite 1800, Philadelphia, Pennsylvania 19103-2899. Accounting and circulation offices: 6277 Sea Harbor Drive, Orlando, FL 32887-4800. Periodicals postage paid at Orlando, FL 32862, and additional mailing offices. Subscription prices are USD 235 per year for US individuals, USD 350 per year for US institutions, USD 115 per year for US students and residents, USD 275 per year for Canadian individuals, USD 430 per year for Canadian institutions, USD 320 per year for international individuals, USD 430 per year for international institutions and USD 155 per year for Canadian and foreign students/residents. To receive student and resident rate, orders must be accompanied by name of affiliated institution, date of term, and the signature of program/residency coordinator on institution letterhead. Orders will be billed at individual rate until proof of status is received. Foreign air speed delivery is included in all Clinics subscription prices. All prices are subject to change without notice. POSTMASTER: Send address changes to *Radiologic Clinics of North America*, W.B. Saunders Company, Periodicals Fulfillment, Orlando, FL 32887-4800. **Customer Service: 1-800-654-2452 (US). From outside of the US, call (+1) 407-345-4000.**

Radiologic Clinics of North America also is published in Greek by Paschalidis Medical Publications, Athens, Greece.

Radiologic Clinics of North America is covered in *Index Medicus, EMBASE/Excerpta Medica, Current Contents/Life Sciences, Current Contents/Clinical Medicine, RSNA Index to Imaging Literature, BIOSIS, Science Citation Index,* and *ISI/BIOMED.*

Printed in the United States of America.

GOAL STATEMENT

The goal of the *Radiologic Clinics of North America* is to keep practicing radiologists and radiology residents up to date with current clinical practice in radiology by providing timely articles reviewing the state of the art in patient care.

ACCREDITATION

The *Radiologic Clinics of North America* is planned and implemented in accordance with the Essential Areas and Policies of the Accreditation Council for Continuing Medical Education (ACCME) through the joint sponsorship of the University of Virginia School of Medicine and Elsevier. The University of Virginia School of Medicine is accredited by the ACCME to provide continuing medical education for physicians.

The University of Virginia School of Medicine designates this educational activity for a maximum of 90 category 1 credits per year, 15 category 1 credits per issue, toward the AMA Physician's Recognition Award. Each physician should claim only those credits that he/she actually spent in the activity.

The American Medical Association has determined that physicians not licensed in the US who participate in this CME activity are eligible for AMA PRA category 1 credit.

AMA PRA category 1 credit can be earned by reading the text material, taking the examination online at *http://www.theclinics.com/home/cme*, and completing the evaluation. After taking the test, your will be required to review any and all incorrect answers. Following completion of the test and the evaluation, your credit will be awarded and you may print your certificate.

FACULTY DISCLOSURE/CONFLICT OF INTEREST

The University of Virginia School of Medicine, as an ACCME accredited provider, endorses and strives to comply with the Accreditation Council for Continuing Medical Education (ACCME) Standards of Commercial Support, Commonwealth of Virginia statutes, University of Virginia policies and procedures, and associated federal and private regulations and guidelines on the need for disclosure and monitoring of proprietary and financial interests that may affect the scientific integrity and balance of content delivered in continuing medical education activities under our auspices.

The University of Virginia School of Medicine requires that all CME activities accredited through this institution be developed independently and be scientifically rigorous, balanced and objective in the presentation/discussion of its content, theories and practices.

All authors/editors participating in an accredited CME activity are expected to disclose to the readers relevant financial relationships with commercial entities occurring within the past 12 months (such as grants or research support, employee, consultant, stock holder, member of speakers bureau, etc.). The University of Virginia School of Medicine will employ appropriate mechanisms to resolve potential conflicts of interest to maintain the standards of fair and balanced education to the reader. Questions about specific strategies can be directed to the Office of Continuing Medical Education, University of Virginia School of Medicine, Charlottesville, Virginia.

The authors/editors listed below have identified no financial or professional relationships for themselves or their spouse/partner:
Linda J. Bagley, MD; Richard A. Bronen, MD; Barton Dudlick, Acquisitions Editor; Adam E. Flanders, MD; Devang M. Gor, MB, BS; P. Ellen Grant, MD; Afshin Karimi, MD, PhD, JD; Jill E. Langer, MD; Laurie A. Loevner, MD; Mahmood F. Mafee, MD, FACR; Robert E. Morales, MD; Mark E. Mullins, MD, PhD; Mark Rapoport, BS; Jay Shah, BS; Jack H. Simon, MD, PhD; M.J.B. Stallmeyer, MD, PhD; Venkatramana R. Vattipally, MD; Ronald L. Wolf, MD, PhD; and David Yu, MD.

The author listed below has not provided disclosures for himself, or spouse/partner:
Sameer A. Ansari, MD, PhD.

Disclosure of Discussion of Non-FDA Approved Uses for Pharmaceutical and/or Medical Devices.
The University of Virginia School of Medicine, as an ACCME provider, requires that all authors identify and disclose any "off label" uses for pharmaceutical and medical device products. The University of Virginia School of Medicine recommends that each physician fully review all the available data on new products or procedures prior to clinical use.

TO ENROLL

To enroll in the Radiologic Clinics of North America Continuing Medical Education program, call customer service at 1-800-654-2452 or sign up online at *http://www.theclinics.com/home/cme.* The CME program is available to subscribers for an additional annual fee USD 205.

THE CLINICS ARE NOW AVAILABLE ONLINE!

Access your subscription at:
www.theclinics.com

NEURORADIOLOGY ESSENTIALS

GUEST EDITOR

RONALD L. WOLF, MD, PhD
Assistant Professor (Radiology), Department of
Neuroradiology, University of Pennsylvania Medical
Center, Philadelphia, Pennsylvania

CONTRIBUTORS

SAMEER A. ANSARI, MD, PhD
Resident, Department of Radiology, University of
Illinois at Chicago Medical Center; and Chief,
Section of Head and Neck Radiology, Department
of Radiology, University of Illinois at Chicago,
Chicago, Illinois

LINDA J. BAGLEY, MD
Associate Professor (Radiology and Neurosurgery),
Department of Radiology, University of
Pennsylvania School of Medicine, University
of Pennsylvania Medical Center, Philadelphia,
Pennsylvania

RICHARD A. BRONEN, MD
Professor, Diagnostic Radiology and Neurosurgery,
Yale University School of Medicine, New Haven,
Connecticut

ADAM E. FLANDERS, MD
Professor (Radiology), Division of
Neuroradiology/ENT, Department of Radiology,
Thomas Jefferson University Hospital,
Philadelphia, Pennsylvania

DEVANG M. GOR, MB, BS
Fellow, Division of Neuroradiology, Department
of Radiology, Hospital of University of
Pennsylvania, University of Pennsylvania Medical
Center, Philadelphia, Pennsylvania

P. ELLEN GRANT, MD
Chief, Division of Pediatric Radiology,
Massachusetts General Hospital, Boston,
Massachusetts

AFSHIN KARIMI, MD, PhD, JD
Resident, Department of Radiology, University of
Illinois Hospital at Chicago, University of Illinois
College of Medicine, Chicago, Illinois

JILL E. LANGER, MD
Associate Professor (Radiology), Division of
Ultrasonography, Department of Radiology,
Hospital of University of Pennsylvania, University
of Pennsylvania Medical Center, Philadelphia,
Pennsylvania

LAURIE A. LOEVNER, MD
Professor (Radiology, Otorhinolaryngology, and
Neurosurgery), Division of Neuroradiology,
Department of Radiology, Hospital of University
of Pennsylvania, University of Pennsylvania
Medical Center, Philadelphia, Pennsylvania

MAHMOOD F. MAFEE, MD, FACR
Medical Director, MRI Center; Professor,
Department of Radiology, University of Illinois at
Chicago Medical Center; and Chief, Section of
Head and Neck Radiology, Department of
Radiology, University of Illinois at Chicago,
Chicago, Illinois

ROBERT E. MORALES, MD
Assistant Professor (Radiology), Division of
Diagnostic and Interventional Neuroradiology,
Department of Diagnostic Radiology, University
of Maryland School of Medicine, Baltimore,
Maryland

MARK E. MULLINS, MD, PhD
Division of Neuroradiology, Massachusetts
General Hospital; and Assistant Professor
(Radiology), Department of Radiology, Harvard
Medical School, Boston, Massachusetts

MARK RAPOPORT, BS
Medical Student, Department of Radiology,
University of Illinois Hospital at Chicago,
University of Illinois College of Medicine,
Chicago, Illinois

JAY SHAH, BS
Medical Student, Department of Radiology,
University of Illinois Hospital at Chicago,
University of Illinois College of Medicine,
Chicago, Illinois

JACK H. SIMON, MD, PhD
Professor (Radiology, Neurology, Neurosurgery,
and Psychiatry); and Vice Chairman (Research),
Department of Radiology, University of Colorado
Health Sciences Center, Denver, Colorado

M.J.B. STALLMEYER, MD, PhD
Assistant Professor (Radiology), Division of
Diagnostic and Interventional Neuroradiology,
Department of Diagnostic Radiology, University
of Maryland School of Medicine, Baltimore,
Maryland

VENKATRAMANA R. VATTIPALLY, MD
Clinical Instructor, Yale University School of
Medicine, New Haven, Connecticut

DAVID YU, MD
Shields MRI Health Care Group, Brockton,
Massachusetts

NEURORADIOLOGY ESSENTIALS

Volume 44 • Number 1 • January 2006

Contents

Approximately 2% to 3% of blunt trauma victims suffer injury to the spinal column each year, often with devastating consequences. This article discusses clinical criteria for screening for spinal injury and the increasing roles of multidetector CT and MR imaging in the evaluation of spinal trauma. Both CT and MR imaging safety issues also are addressed. Lastly, the role of imaging in the evaluation of whiplash injury, instability, vascular injury, and delayed traumatic sequelae is discussed.

Traumatic injury to the major vessels of the head and neck can result in potentially devastating neurologic sequelae. Until recently, conventional angiography was the primary imaging modality used to evaluate these often challenging patients. Advances in cross-sectional imaging have improved the ability to screen for these lesions, which have been found to be more common than previously thought; however, accepted protocols of imaging evaluation have not yet been fully established. This article presents a general approach to the patient with suspected neurovascular injury. This includes a discussion of the histopathologic spectrum, clinical presentation, mechanisms, radiologic work-up, pertinent issues of the most common lesions, and some of the endovascular techniques used in their management.

Stroke remains one of the most important clinical diagnoses for which patients are referred to the radiologist for emergent imaging. Timely and accurate imaging guides admission from the emergency department or transfer to a hospital with a dedicated stroke service, triage to the intensive care unit, anticoagulation, thrombolysis, and many other forms of treatment and management. It is important to approach each patient's imaging needs logically and tailor each work-up, and constantly to review the entire process for potential improvements. Time saved in getting an accurate diagnosis of stroke may indeed decrease morbidity and mortality. This article discusses the current management of stroke imaging and reviews the relevant literature.

Acute Injury to the Immature Brain with Hypoxia with or Without Hypoperfusion   63

P. Ellen Grant and David Yu

This article reviews the imaging features and evolution of immature brain injury caused by hypoxia with or without hypoperfusion in the neonate and young child. Clinical presentations and available literature on mechanisms and clinical outcomes are discussed. In many of these cases, diffusion-weighted imaging does not show the full extent of the injury but detects a pattern of injury that is important in guiding clinical care. Awareness of the delayed cell death mechanisms is essential to understand diffusion-weighted imaging sensitivity and evolution and to provide the most accurate clinical interpretation, especially in cases of hypoxia with or without hypoperfusion.

Update on Multiple Sclerosis   79

Jack H. Simon

In this article the basic features of the focal MR imaging lesions and the underlying pathology are reviewed. Next, the diffuse pathology in the normal-appearing white and gray matter as revealed by conventional and quantitative MR imaging techniques is discussed, including reference to how the focal and diffuse pathology may be in part linked through axonal-neuronal degeneration. The MR imaging criteria incorporated for the first time into formal clinical diagnostic criteria for multiple sclerosis are next discussed. Finally, a discussion is provided as to how MR imaging is used in monitoring subclinical disease either before or subsequent to initiation of treatment, in identifying aggressive subclinical disease, and in monitoring treatment.

Imaging of Cervical Lymph Nodes in Head and Neck Cancer: The Basics   101

Devang M. Gor, Jill E. Langer, and Laurie A. Loevner

Imaging can identify pathologic cervical adenopathy in a significant number of patients with head and neck cancer who have no palpable adenopathy on physical examination. This article reviews nodal classification, drainage patterns of different head and neck cancers, various cross-sectional imaging features of metastatic lymph nodes from head and neck cancer, nodal staging, and certain features like extracapsular spread and carotid and vertebral invasion that the radiologist should know because they have therapeutic and prognostic implications. New imaging techniques and the role of fluorodeoxyglucose positron emission tomography imaging in recurrent disease are discussed.

Special Articles

MR Imaging of Epilepsy: Strategies for Successful Interpretation   111

Venkatramana R. Vattipally and Richard A. Bronen

The first half of this article is devoted to providing an introduction and overview for MR imaging of epilepsy. Several MR imaging epilepsy topics will be discussed in great detail in separate articles, such as hippocampal sclerosis, developmental disorders, and functional MR imaging. The remainder of this review will discuss strategies for successful interpretation of MR images from the seizure patiet and how to avoid potential pitfalls.

ELSEVIER
SAUNDERS

RADIOLOGIC
CLINICS
OF NORTH AMERICA

Radiol Clin N Am 44 (2006) xi

Preface
Neuroradiology Essentials

Ronald L. Wolf, MD, PhD
Guest Editor

Department of Neuroradiology
University of Pennsylvania Medical Center
3400 Spruce Street
Philadelphia, PA 19104, USA

E-mail address:
ronald.wolf@uphs.upenn.edu

When asked to serve as the Guest Editor for an issue of *Radiologic Clinics of North America* including essential neuroradiology topics, I decided to focus on some of the most common conditions in which imaging plays a key role. Although common—or rather, because they are common—advances in treatment and management strategies as well as imaging strategies make it necessary to constantly reassess our understanding and approach to these problems. The goal of this issue was to provide a practical approach to each problem, incorporating relevant clinical and radiologic advances.

Trauma is unfortunately all too common, and this is the topic of the first two articles. Over the last several years, cross-sectional imaging requests from our trauma services have been increasing quite steeply, at least partially due to the proliferation of multidetector CT scanners and the wealth of information available with this technique. In the first article, traumatic injury to the spinal column is discussed. This is followed by an article discussing the imaging of neurovascular traumatic injury. Screening for such injuries has become much more aggressive, and yet, widely accepted guidelines for screening are not fully established. In the next two articles, the focus is on the most common

mechanisms of nontraumatic brain injury in the adult and pediatric populations: ischemic injury in adults and hypoxic injury with or without hypoperfusion for children. These types of injury can certainly occur in both populations, but the etiologies and resulting patterns and mechanisms of injury are quite different. The next two articles thus focus on adult and pediatric populations separately. In the outpatient setting, two of the most common imaging requests are for cervical node evaluation and multiple sclerosis. These are the topics for the next two articles. Finally, for the benefit of the reader, two additional articles relevant to essential neuroradiology and previously published in *Neuroimaging Clinics of North America* have been included: one providing an overview of epilepsy and a discussion of MR imaging interpretation in this setting, and the other reviewing imaging of orbital pathology.

I am of course indebted to the authors for taking time out of their busy schedules to provide comprehensive and practical discussions of these topics. I would also like to express my gratitude to the series editor, Mr. Barton Dudlick, for his guidance and remarkable patience in the preparation of this issue.

0033-8389/06/$ – see front matter © 2005 Elsevier Inc. All rights reserved.
radiologic.theclinics.com

doi:10.1016/j.rcl.2005.10.005

RADIOLOGIC
CLINICS
OF NORTH AMERICA

Radiol Clin N Am 44 (2006) 1–12

Imaging of Spinal Trauma

Linda J. Bagley, MD*

- Indications for imaging
- Cervical spine imaging
- Thoracic and lumbar imaging
- Concerns about radiation dosing
- Screening of pediatric patients
- MR imaging
- Clinical issues
  Instability

Whiplash
Vascular injury
Subacute and chronic injuries
- Summary
- References

Approximately 30,000 injuries to the spinal column occur in the United States each year. Most injuries are secondary to blunt trauma (motor vehicle accidents, falls, sports injuries), although penetrating trauma accounts for approximately 10% to 20% of the cases. Roughly 2% to 3% of blunt trauma victims are affected, with the incidence of cervical spinal trauma being increased in those with significant craniofacial trauma. Approximately 40% to 50% of spinal injuries produce a neurologic deficit, often severe and sometimes fatal [1]. Survival is inversely correlated with patient age, and mortality during initial hospitalization approaches 10% [2]. Because most patients affected are young, the costs of lifetime care and rehabilitation are extremely high, often exceeding $1,000,000 per individual [3]. Plain radiography, CT, and MR imaging may all be used in the evaluation of the spinal column and are often complementary.

Indications for imaging

Pain, neurologic deficit, distracting injuries, altered consciousness (caused by head injury, intoxication, or pharmaceutical intervention), and high-risk mechanism of injury have been shown to be appropriate, highly sensitive clinical indications for spinal imaging. In the multicenter National Emergency X-Radiography Use Study led by Hoffman and coworkers [4], 34,069 blunt trauma patients underwent cervical spine imaging, 4309 (12.6%) of whom did not meet the clinical criteria for imaging discussed previously. A total of 818 injuries were reported in this study, eight occurring in the group that would not otherwise have been imaged. Two of those injuries were clinically significant. Overall sensitivity for clinical evaluation was approximately 99.6%. Similarly, the Canadian C-Spine Rule study identified patients judged to be "low risk" (ambulatory, without midline tenderness or immediate onset of pain, able to attain a sitting position, victims of simple rear-end motor vehicle crashes). Such low-risk patients who could actively turn their heads 45 degrees in both directions were deemed not to require imaging. Overall sensitivity of clinical criteria in this study was 100% [5]. Similar clinical criteria have been evaluated in the thoracic and lumbar spine. Frankel and coworkers

Department of Radiology, University of Pennsylvania School of Medicine, University of Pennsylvania Medical Center, Philadelphia, PA, USA
* Department of Radiology, University of Pennsylvania School of Medicine, University of Pennsylvania Medical Center, 3400 Spruce Street, Philadelphia, PA 19104.
E-mail address: linda.bagley@uphs.upenn.edu

doi:10.1016/j.rcl.2005.08.004
radiologic.theclinics.com

[6] reported 100% sensitivity when the clinical criteria of back pain, the presence of a neurologic deficit, a Glasgow Coma Scale score of 8 or less, a fall from a height of 10 feet or more, ejection from a motorcycle, or involvement in a motor vehicle accident with speeds greater than 50 miles per hour were applied.

Cervical spine imaging

In the setting of acute spinal trauma, CT scanning has been shown to be more time efficient [7,8] and significantly more sensitive for fracture detection than plain films [9–16]. Multidetector CT provides superior evaluation of bony anatomy and pathol-

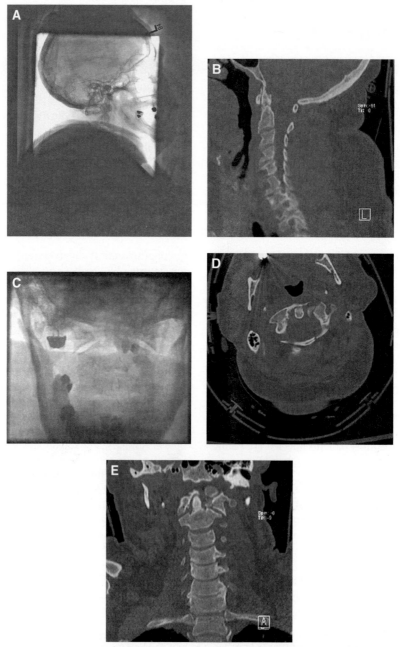

Fig. 1. (*A*) Lateral plain film is quite limited, imaging only to C2, demonstrating irregularity and possible fractures of C2. (*B*) Sagittal reformatted view reveals a fracture through the base of the odontoid. (*C*) Open mouth odontoid view demonstrates lateral displacement of the lateral masses of C1. (*D* and *E*) Axial CT scan and coronal reformatted view reveal a markedly comminuted fracture of the atlas with lateral displacement of the left lateral mass.

ogy. Images may be rapidly acquired and reconstructed at narrow intervals (eg, 1 mm) with edge-enhancing algorithms. Multiplanar and three-dimensional images can subsequently be created [**Fig. 1**]. In a number of studies, the sensitivity of CT scanning for cervical spinal fracture detection has been reported to be between 90% and 99% with specificities of 72% to 89%. In contrast, the reported sensitivity of plain films has ranged from 39% to 94% with variable specificity. Sensitivity of plain films has inversely correlated with severity of trauma sustained [9–16]. Multiple studies have demonstrated the limitations of plain radiography in the cervical spine, particularly at the craniocervical and cervicothoracic junctions. In a 1995 study by Link and coworkers [17], patients with substantial head trauma (Glasgow Coma Scale 3–6) underwent axial CT scanning of the craniocervical junction. Eighteen percent of patients had fractures of C1, C2, or occipital condyles. Eight of nine occipital condyle fractures and 13 of 33 fractures of C1 or C2 were not seen on plain films. Although most condylar fractures are stable, these injuries may be a cause of persistent pain, produce cranial nerve deficits, or lead to vertebrobasilar vascular injury or compromise [**Fig. 2**]. Furthermore, 6 of 13 fractures of C1 or C2 seen on CT only were unstable. Similarly, Nunez and coworkers [18] compared lateral plain films with helical CT of the cervical spine performed with 5-mm collimation and sagittal and coronal reformatted images. Thirty-two of 88 fractures detected by CT were not seen on limited plain film evaluation, and one third of those fractures were clinically significant or unstable.

In addition, a number of centers have reported CT scanning in moderate- to high-risk trauma patients to be a more cost-effective screening mo-dality than plain radiography when the costs of missed injuries and preventable paralysis (including the costs of prolonged hospitalizations, rehabilitation, lost productivity, and malpractice suits) are taken into account [10,11]. Delays in diagnoses of clinically significant cervical spine injuries have been reported in approximately 5% to 23% of patients in various series, most of which used plain radiography as the initial screening modality. Neurologic deterioration (possibly secondary to mismanagement) occurred in 10% to 50% of these patients [19]. In contrast, development of a secondary neurologic deficit occurred in only 1.4% of patients whose injuries were detected on initial screening in Reid and coworkers' cohort [20]. CT is rapidly becoming the initial screening modality for osseous spinal pathology in adults, particularly those judged to be at moderate to high risk for spinal fracture based on mechanism of injury and clinical data.

Thoracic and lumbar imaging

Thoracic and lumbar spinal injuries also affect approximately 2% to 3% of blunt trauma victims and are associated with an approximately 40% to 50% incidence of neurologic deficit. CT scanning has been shown to be superior to plain films for detection and characterization of fractures. In a 1995 study by Campbell and coworkers [21], 20% of unstable burst fractures (involving the posterior vertebral body cortex) of the thoracic and lumbar spine were misdiagnosed as stable wedge compression fractures (single-column injuries) by plain films. CT better detected fractures of the posterior elements, malalignment, and intracanalicular fragments. Given the frequency with which many vic-

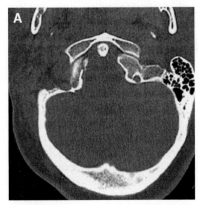
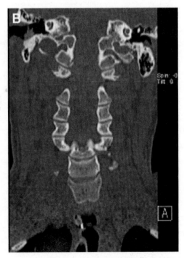

Fig. 2. (*A* and *B*) Axial and coronal reformatted CT scans demonstrate a mildly displaced fracture of the right occipital condyle.

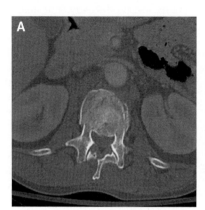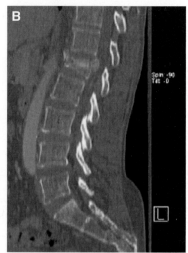

Fig. 3. (A) Axial reconstructed CT image reveals a comminuted burst fracture of L1 with retropulsed posterior cortex and a large prevertebral hematoma. (B) Sagittal reformatted view demonstrates marked loss of height of the vertebral body with retropulsed cortex and canal compromise.

tims of blunt trauma undergo multidetector CT scanning of the chest, abdomen, and pelvis, the use of reformatted images from visceral protocol CT scans to evaluate the spine has dramatically increased [Fig. 3] [22–25]. When compared with plain radiography in the study by Sheridan and coworkers [22], visceral CT scans reformatted at 2.5-mm intervals with sagittal and coronal reconstructed views were shown to improve sensitivity for detection of lumbar fractures from 95% to 97% and of thoracic fractures from 62% to 86%. Detail and likely sensitivity can be further improved with reformatting performed at 1-mm intervals.

Concerns about radiation dosing

Although CT scanning has been shown to be more time efficient and in certain circumstances more cost effective than plain radiography, there is a significant increase in radiation exposure associated with CT screening [26,27]. Adelgeis and coworkers [28] reported an approximately 50% increase in mean radiation dose to the cervical spine in pediatric patients for helical CT compared with conventional radiography. When organ-specific doses were examined, the results were even more concerning. Rybicki and coworkers [29] found an approximately 10-fold increase in radiation dose to the skin (28 versus 2.89 mGy) and an approximately 14-fold increase in dose to the thyroid (26 versus 1.80 mGy) with CT examination of the entire cervical spine (using 3-mm collimation, pitch of 1.5:1, 120 kV [peak], and 240 mA and single lateral radiograph) rather than a four- to five-view radiographic series.

Screening of pediatric patients

Spinal injuries in children occur somewhat less commonly than in adults, with pediatric spinal injuries accounting for approximately 2% to 5% of all such injuries. The types of injuries sustained in children, particularly younger children (under age 8), also differ from those sustained in adults. Mechanisms of injury often differ with age. The upper cervical spine is most often affected in children, and dislocations and cord injuries without associated fractures occur more often in children than in adults [30,31]. Furthermore, the tissues and organs of children, particularly those under age 5, are more prone to development of radiation-induced malignancies, because of increased radiosensitivity of certain organs; a longer expected lifetime in which to develop a cancer; and frequent failure of adjustment of scanning parameters (eg, tube current) based on patient size [26]. Multiple series have demonstrated little improvement in detection of fractures and malalignment with CT compared with plain films in the pediatric population [28,32], with substantial increases in radiation exposure reported with CT. Many normal anatomic variants in children, however, may mimic fractures and warrant additional evaluation with CT or MR imaging [33]. Because children often require sedation for CT scanning, the improvements in time efficiency and length of emergency department stay observed in adults undergoing CT screening are often not appreciated in children [32]. Given these differences between children and adults, spinal trauma screening protocols must be modified for the pediatric population. Plains films may be used as the initial screening modality with CT

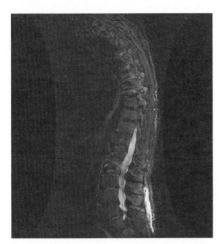

Fig. 4. Sagittal STIR image is notable for compression deformities of the T12 through L2 vertebrae. Marrow edema is present within L2, indicative of fracture acuity.

scans limited to areas of interest. Reductions in tube current and increases in table and gantry rotation speeds may be used to reduce radiation exposure [26,34]. MR imaging has a larger role in the evaluation of pediatric spinal trauma because of the increased incidence of spinal cord injury without radiographic abnormality.

MR imaging

MR imaging, with superior tissue characterization, provides the best evaluation of soft tissue pathology and essentially the only direct evaluation of the spinal cord [3]. Information obtained regarding disks, ligaments, hematomas, and the spinal cord is often complementary to the evaluation of osseous pathology provided by CT scanning [3]. MR imaging with STIR or fat-saturated T2-weighted sequences may also detect additional regions of bone edema and aid in the determination of acuity of osseous injuries [Fig. 4]. MR imaging is indicated in the setting of spinal trauma when a neurologic deficit is present or when there is clinical suspicion of a soft tissue or vascular abnormality. High-resolution, heavily T2-weighted sequences can be used (as an alternative to myelography) for the detection of potential nerve root avulsions and pseudomeningocele formation [Fig. 5]. MR imaging may also be used to evaluate posttraumatic sequelae, such as myelomalacia, syrinx formation, cord tethering, and development of arteriovenous fistulas.

Many safety considerations arise when performing MR imaging in trauma victims with suspected spinal injury. Many such patients are critically ill and require extensive monitoring and ventilatory support. Ventilators and pulse, blood pressure, and oxygenation monitors must be MR imaging compatible. Spinal precautions must be maintained at all times. Fixation devices, such as halos, may be fitted with MR imaging–compatible vests that contain graphite, thereby minimizing image degradation. Traction devices may impede table motion and may prove a danger to the patient and the MR imaging personnel, should they become projectiles [35]. Additional concerns arise in patients who have suffered penetrating trauma with retained metallic fragments [36,37]. The practice of imaging patients with retained spinal bullets is controversial. Most firearm ammunition is nonferrous but rarely is the composition of the retained projectile known. At least theoretically, a ferrous fragment may become mobile in the magnetic field and produce additional neurologic damage. Multiple small case series have, however, reported no adverse affects in patients with bullets within or in proximity to the spinal canal. In many of these

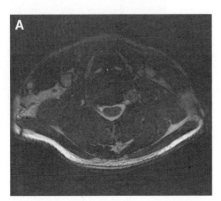
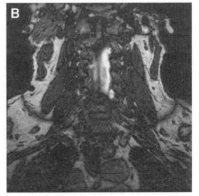

Fig. 5. (*A* and *B*) Axial and coronal high-resolution heavily T2-weighted images (FIESTA sequence) reveal a small pseudomeningocele in the left neural foramen and absence of the traversing nerve root, indicative of a nerve root avulsion.

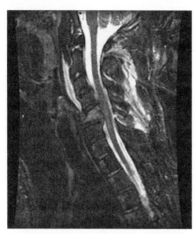

Fig. 6. Sagittal STIR image demonstrates an acute compression fracture of C5 with extensive bone edema and retropulsion, resulting in effacement of the ventral cerebrospinal fluid space. There is abnormal signal intensity within the cord with associated expansion, representing contusion, extending from C4 through C7. There is also a large prevertebral hematoma, and there is extensive signal abnormality within the interspinous ligaments and posterior paraspinal musculature.

cases, management was altered by the MR imaging findings [38].

Canal and foraminal compromise and cord compression, in the presence or absence of acute fracture, are well evaluated with MR imaging. Spondylotic changes, disk herniations, and epidural and subdural hematomas may all narrow the canal and neural foramina. Thin-section T2-weighted gradient echo images provide optimal evaluation of degenerative changes. T2-weighted images can best detect areas of cord signal abnormality, representing contusion and adversely effecting patient prognosis [Fig. 6] [3,39].

Ligamentous and soft tissue injuries are best detected on fat-saturated T2-weighted images. The normal anterior and posterior longitudinal ligaments are seen as continuous, thin, hypointense structures along the ventral and dorsal surfaces of the vertebral bodies on sagittal images. The ligamenta flava and intraspinous ligaments may also be directly evaluated. When injury has occurred, focal areas of increased T2-weighted signal intensity or frank discontinuities in the ligaments may be seen [Fig. 7] [3,39].

Clinical issues

Instability

Stability of the cervical spine is best assessed with a functional examination that includes flexion and extension views. Such an examination, however,

should be reserved for alert, cooperative patients with a normal neurologic examination and without radiographic evidence of injuries that are almost certainly unstable. Because of pain and muscle spasm present at the time of acute injury, patient motion is often limited. As such, delayed flexion and extension views (obtained 7–10 days following the injury) may be more informative. Instability is diagnosed when there is more than 3.5-mm horizontal displacement between the flexion and extension positions. Other findings suggestive of instability include displaced apophyseal joints, widened disk spaces, loss of over 30% of the vertebral body height, and the presence of a prevertebral hematoma. For those patients not suitable for flexion and extension radiography, MR imaging can be obtained. MR imaging directly images the ligaments and soft tissues of the cervical spine and can be used to infer stability or instability in such patients [39].

Whiplash

Whiplash injuries are exceedingly common, frequently following rear-end motor vehicle accidents with hyperflexion and hyperextension of the neck. Reported symptoms include neck pain or stiffness, paresthesias, upper extremity pain, jaw pain, and headaches. Recovery is often somewhat delayed, taking weeks or months. Most patients, however, report resolution of symptoms within a year of the injury; in the Quebec Task Force study, 97% of such patients reported resolution of symptoms, although 10% to 42% of patients in other studies have reported the development of chronic neck pain [40–42]. The etiology of whiplash symptoms

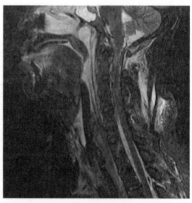

Fig. 7. Sagittal STIR image demonstrates extensive soft tissue and ligamentous injury with increased signal intensity throughout the posterior paraspinal musculature, interspinous ligaments, and prevertebral space. A distraction injury at C1-2 was suspected and verified on additional sequences and on CT. There is signal abnormality at the pontomedullary junction and within the spinal cord at C2.

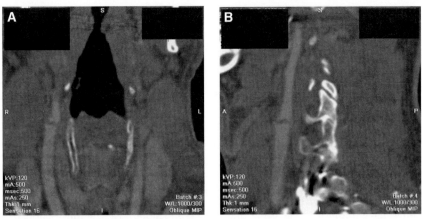

Fig. 8. Coronal (*A*) and sagittal (*B*) reformatted maximal intensity projections reveal a linear defect in the proximal right internal carotid artery. This was a blunt injury (struck in neck by hockey puck).

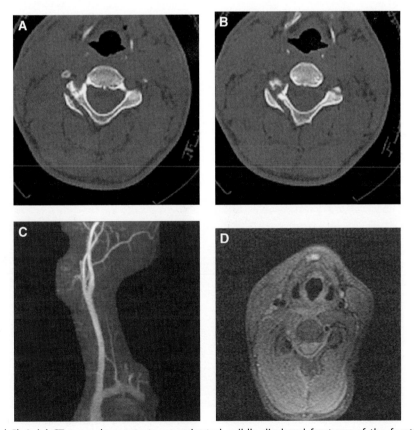

Fig. 9. (*A* and *B*) Axial CT scans demonstrate comminuted, mildly displaced fractures of the facet joints and a fracture of the right pedicle extending into the foramen transversarium. (*C*) Two-dimensional time-of-flight MR angiography demonstrates occlusion of the right vertebral artery in its midcervical portion. (*D*) Axial fat-saturated T1-weighted image at the level of the facet fractures does not reveal a flow void in the right vertebral artery. Hyperintensity within the right vertebral artery likely represents thrombus. There is surrounding signal abnormality, hematoma, indicative of dissection.

and the role of imaging in their evaluation remain controversial. Proposed causes include muscle tears; ligamentous injuries; apophyseal joint injuries; temporomandibular joint injuries; discogenic disease; perineural scarring; and facet, pillar, end plate, or vertebral body fractures. In the acutely injured patient with whiplash, Ronnen and coworkers [43] have suggested that imaging is not cost effective. In their study of 100 such patients who underwent MR imaging within 3 weeks of injury, only 1 had an abnormality directly attributable to the trauma. Similar findings were reported by Borchgrevink and coworkers [44] in a group of 40 patients studied within 2 days of injury. Many additional studies have found imaging, other than

initial screening, to be of limited value [45]. Imaging is, however, more likely to play a role in the evaluation of the persistently symptomatic patient. Jonsson and coworkers [46] did find eight acute disk herniations in 24 patients who had neck pain for 6 weeks or more following injury. Management strategies are even more controversial [41]. Steroids, analgesics, soft collars, immobilization, activity limitation, physical therapy, exercise, radiofrequency neurotomies, acupuncture, diskectomies, fusion procedures, and steroid, botulinum toxin, and anesthetic injections have all been used. Many have been shown to be of limited or no benefit. In small, often uncontrolled series, high-dose methylprednisolone given within 8 hours of injury has

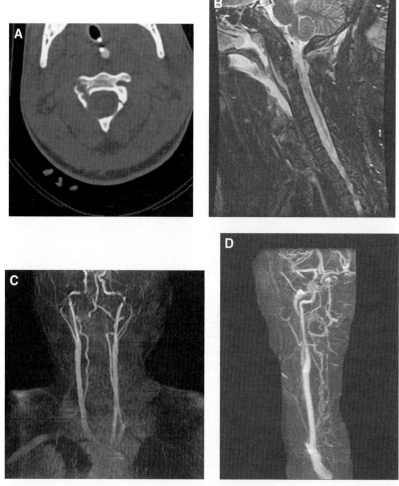

Fig. 10. (*A*) Axial CT scan demonstrates a fracture of C2 extending through the right foramen transversarium and left lamina. (*B*) Sagittal T2-weighted MR image is notable for a mildly displaced fracture of C2 with edema at the fracture site and a large amount of prevertebral soft tissue swelling. (*C*) Two-dimensional time-of-flight MR angiogram reveals marked irregularity of the right vertebral artery at the C1-2 level. (*D*) Gadolinium-enhanced three-dimensional time-of-flight MR angiography is notable for extensive venous opacification, predominantly within the spinal canal, secondary to a vertebrovenous fistula, subsequently confirmed on conventional angiography.

been shown to reduce sick leave, active exercise has been shown to reduce somatic complaints, and trigger point injections with botulinum toxin have provided short-term pain reduction [41]. Radiofrequency neurotomies and intra-articular local anesthetic injections have been shown in multiple studies to improve patient symptomatology, particularly neck pain and headache [41].

Vascular injury

The incidence of vascular injury in all victims of blunt trauma is less than 1%. It is substantially higher, however, in certain subsets of patients deemed high risk [47–51]. The incidence of vertebral arterial injury following major blunt cervical spinal trauma has been estimated to be as high as 24% to 46%; most of these lesions are, however, asymptomatic [48–50]. Screening for vascular injury is indicated in patients with otherwise unexplained neurologic deficits; in patients who sustained hyperextension and hyperflexion injuries; and in those with severe blunt trauma to the neck (including that produced by seat belts) [Fig. 8]. Other indications for screening include cervical spine or skull base fractures (particularly those adjacent to or involving vascular foramina), and penetrating injuries adjacent to vascular structures [47–51]. Multiple modalities have been used for detection, evaluation, or treatment of vascular injuries [52–55]. In the absence of contraindications, MR imaging and MR angiography may be used for optimal detection of mural hematoma and dissection [Fig. 9] [52]. Pseudoaneurysms may be present at the time of injury or may develop following

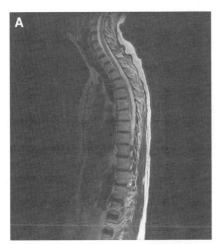
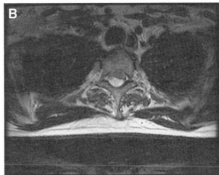
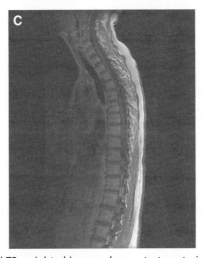

Fig. 11. (*A* and *B*) Sagittal and axial T2-weighted images demonstrate anterior and left lateral displacement and compression of the upper thoracic cord by an intradural extramedullary lesion with signal intensity characteristics of cerebrospinal fluid (an arachnoid cyst, likely resulting from adhesions in the subarachnoid space). This could alternatively represent adhesion/cord tethering/cord herniation. (*C*) Gadolinium-enhanced sagittal T1-weighted image reveals no pathologic enhancement.

dissections. Pseudoaneurysms and arteriovenous fistulae may also be detected with MR imaging and MR angiography, but are optimally studied with conventional angiography. Traumatic vertebral arteriovenous fistulae most often occur in the lower cervical spine and may produce various neurologic and nonneurologic symptoms, including pulsatile tinnitus; neck pain; dizziness and syncope (caused by steal phenomena); and paralysis [**Fig. 10**]. In cases of penetrating trauma in stable patients, CT and CT angiography may be superior for detection of direct puncture injury and for delineation of trajectory of the penetrating instrument [53,54]. Retained metallic fragments may, however, degrade such studies. Conventional angiography with potential for endovascular therapy is certainly warranted in cases of active hemorrhage, new-onset cerebral ischemia in patients without contraindications to thrombolysis, suspected arteriovenous fistulae, expanding pseudoaneurysms, and when noninvasive modalities have been inconclusive [47–51].

Subacute and chronic injuries

Although some patients recover some neurologic function in the months and years following injury, others suffer progressive neurologic deterioration. Worsening myelopathy, ascending neurologic level, worsening pain, worsening sensory deficit, increased spasticity, and autonomic dysfunction may occur. Possible etiologies include myelomalacia, syrinx formation, continued or progressive cord compression, instability, and development of adhesions with associated cord tethering [56]. Adhesions and tethering may be suggested when loculated collections of cerebrospinal fluid are seen and when the cord appears abnormal in course, position, or configuration (caused by compression) [**Fig. 11**]. The imaging appearance of myelomalacia is that of ill-defined signal abnormality with associated cord atrophy Cystic myelomalacia is often associated with chronic or recurrent cord compression. Microcysts may initially develop in areas of prior hemorrhage, demyelination, or ischemia. These microcysts may coalesce, and syrinx formation may ultimately result [**Fig. 12**]. On MR imaging, signal-intensity characteristics of the syrinx cavity typically follow those of cerebrospinal fluid, although they may differ if proteinaceous fluid is present. Additionally, the spinal cord appears focally expanded. In patients with previous spinal cord injuries and new neurologic deficits, syrinx formation is common. Symptomatic intramedullary cysts or syrinx cavities may be treated with surgical drainage or shunting [3,39].

Vascular injury was discussed in greater detail previously, and is the topic of a more focused

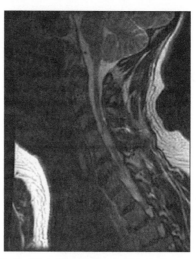

Fig. 12. Sagittal T2-weighted image demonstrates cystic myelomalacia of the cord at C4 and C5. There has been fusion of the C4 and C5 vertebrae. A disk-osteophyte complex is present at C6–7.

discussion elsewhere in this issue. Briefly, arterial dissections, transections, and arteriovenous fistulae may occur at the time of injury with progression or regression of luminal compromise, development and enlargement of pseudoaneurysms, and development of venous hypertension over time. MR imaging and MR angiography may directly image the vascular pathology or reveal indirect signs of it, such as cerebral infarction resulting from dissections or pseudoaneurysms or cord swelling and enlarged pial veins seen with arteriovenous fistulae.

Summary

Spinal trauma often has devastating consequences. Well-controlled clinical trials have established guidelines for appropriate use of imaging and clinically based screening. As technology has evolved, multidetector CT scanning has assumed a significant role as a primary screening modality, although radiologists and clinicians must be conscious of the increased radiation dose that accompanies it, particularly when children are being imaged. MR imaging is often a complementary examination, providing improved soft tissue detail of the spinal cord, disks, and ligaments. Vascular injuries have been increasingly recognized in association with spinal trauma, and MR angiography, CT angiography, and conventional angiography all have roles in their detection and possible treatment. Lastly, patients with spinal injuries may suffer progressive neurologic deterioration, and imaging again has a role in their diagnosis and management.

References

[1] Hills MW, Dean SA. Head injury and facial injury: is there an increased risk of cervical spine injury? J Trauma 1993;34:549–54.

[2] Pope AM, Tarlov AR. Disability in America: toward a national agenda for prevention. Washington: National Academy Press; 1991.

[3] Flanders AE, Croul SE. Spinal trauma. In: Atlas SW, editor. Magnetic resonance imaging of the brain and spine. 3rd edition. Philadelphia: Lippincott, Williams, and Wilkins; 2002. p. 1769–824.

[4] Hoffman JR, Mower WR, Wolfson AB, et al. Validity of a set of clinical criteria to rule out injury to the cervical spine in patients with blunt trauma. National Emergency X-Radiography Utilization Study Group. N Engl J Med 2000;343: 94–9.

[5] Stiell IG, Wells GA, Vandemheen KL, et al. The Canadian C-spine rule for radiography in alert and stable trauma patients. JAMA 2001;286: 1841–8.

[6] Frankel HL, Rozycki GS, Ochsner MG, et al. Indications for obtaining surveillance thoracic and lumbar spine radiographs. J Trauma 1994; 37:673–6.

[7] Daffner RH. Cervical radiography for trauma patients: a time-effective technique? AJR Am J Roentgenol 2000;175:1309–11.

[8] Daffner RH. Helical CT of the cervical spine for trauma patients: a time study. AJR Am J Roentgenol 2001;177:677–9.

[9] Widder S, Doig C, Burrowes P, et al. Prospective evaluation of computed tomographic scanning for spinal clearance of obtunded trauma patients: preliminary results. J Trauma 2004;56: 1179–84.

[10] Blackmore CC, Ramsey SD, Mann FA, et al. Cervical spine screening with CT in trauma patients: a cost effectiveness analysis. Radiology 1999;212: 117–25.

[11] Grogan EL, Morris JA, Dittus RS, et al. Cervical spine evaluation in urban trauma centers: lowering institutional costs and complications through helical CT scan. J Am Coll Surg 2005; 200:160–5.

[12] Brandt MM, Wahl WL, Yoem K, et al. Computed tomographic scanning reduces cost and time of complete spine evaluation. J Trauma 2004;56: 1022–8.

[13] Tins BJ, Cessar-Pullicino VN. Imaging of acute cervical spine injuries: review and outlook. Clin Radiol 2004;59:865–80.

[14] Blackmore CC, Mann FA, Wilson AJ. Helical CT in the primary trauma evaluation of the cervical spine: an evidence based approach. Skeletal Radiol 2000;29:632–9.

[15] Schenarts PJ, Diaz J, Kaiser C, et al. Prospective comparison of admission computed tomographic scan and plain films of the upper cervical spine in trauma patients with altered mental status. J Trauma 2001;51:663–8.

[16] Nguyen GK, Clark R. Adequacy of plain radiography in the diagnosis if cervical spine injuries. Emerg Radiol 2005;11(3):158–61.

[17] Link TM, Schuierer G, Hufendiek A, et al. Substantial head trauma: value of routine CT examination of the cervicocranium. Radiology 1995; 196:741–5.

[18] Nunez DB, Zuluaga A, Fuentes-Bernardo DA, et al. Cervical spine trauma: how much more do we learn routinely by using helical CT? Radiographics 1996;16:1307–18.

[19] Poonnoose PM, Ravichandran F, McClelland MR. Missed and mismanaged injuries of the spinal cord. J Trauma 2002;53:314–20.

[20] Reid DC, Henderson R, Saboe L, et al. Etiology and clinical course of missed spine fractures. J Trauma 1987;27:980–6.

[21] Campbell SE, Phillips CD, Dubovsky E, et al. The value of CT in determining potential instability of simple wedge-compression fractures of the lumbar spine. AJNR Am J Neuroradiol 1995;16: 1385–92.

[22] Sheridan R, Peralta R, Rhea J, et al. Reformatted visceral protocol helical computed tomographic scanning allows conventional radiographs of the thoracic and lumbar spine to be eliminated in the evaluation of blunt trauma patients. J Trauma 2003;55:665–9.

[23] Roos JE, Hilfiker P, Platz A, et al. MDCT in emergency radiology: is a standardized chest of abdominal protocol sufficient for evaluation of thoracic and lumbar spine trauma? AJR Am J Roentgenol 2004;183:959–68.

[24] Watura R, Cobby M, Taylor J. Multislice CT in imaging of trauma of the spine, pelvis, and complex foot injuries. Br J Radiol 2004;77: 46–63.

[25] Herzog C, Ahle H, Mack MG, et al. Traumatic injuries of the pelvis and thoracic and lumbar spine: does thin-slice multidetector-row CT increase diagnostic accuracy? Eur Radiol 2004;14: 1751–60.

[26] Frush DP, Donnelly LF, Rosen NS. Computed tomography and radiation risks: what pediatric health care providers should know. Pediatrics 2003;112:951–7.

[27] Frush DP. Review of radiation issues for computed tomography. Semin Ultrasound CT MR 2004;25:15–24.

[28] Adelgais KM, Grossman DC, Langer SG, et al. Use of helical computed tomography for imaging the pediatric cervical spine. Acad Emerg Med 2004;11:228–36.

[29] Rybicki F, Nawfel RD, Judy PF, et al. Skin and thyroid dosimetry in cervical spine screening: two methods for evaluation and a comparison between a helical CT and radiographic trauma series. AJR Am J Roentgenol 2002;179: 933–7.

[30] Hamilton MG, Myles ST. Pediatric spinal injury: review of 174 hospital admissions. J Neurosurg 1992;77:700–4.

[31] Brown RL, Brunn MA, Garcia VF. Cervical spine injuries in children: a review of 103 patients treated consecutively at a level 1 pediatric trauma center. J Pediatr Surg 2001;36:1107–14.

[32] Hernandez JA, Chupik C, Swischuk LE. Cervical spine trauma in children under 5 years: productivity of CT. Emerg Radiol 2004;10:176–8.

[33] Avellino AM, Mann FA, Grady MS, et al. The misdiagnosis of acute cervical spine injuries and fractures in infants and children: the 12-year experience of a level 1 pediatric and adult trauma center. Childs Nerv Syst 2005;21:122–7.

[34] Kalra MK, Mahar MM, Rizzo S, et al. Radiation exposure and projected risks with multidetector-row computed tomographic scanning: clinical strategies and technologic developments for dose reduction. J Comput Assist Tomogr 2004; 28(Suppl 1):S46–9.

[35] Shellock FG. MR imaging and cervical fixation devices: evaluation of ferromagnetism, heating and artifacts at 1.5 tesla. Magn Reson Imaging 1996;14:1093–8.

[36] Smith AS, Hurst GC, Duerk JL, et al. MR of ballistic materials: imaging artifacts and potential hazards. AJNR Am J Neuroradiol 1991; 12:567–72.

[37] Teitelbaum GP, Yee CA, Van Horn DD, et al. Metallic ballistic fragments: MR imaging safety and artifacts. Radiology 1990;175:855–9.

[38] Smugar SS, Schweitzer ME, Hume E. MRI in patients with intraspinal bullets. J Magn Reson Imaging 1999;9:151–3.

[39] Bagley LJ. MR of spinal trauma. In: Taveras JM, Ferrucci JT, editors. Radiology: diagnosis, imaging, intervention. Philadelphia: Lippincott, Williams, and Wilkins; 2002. p. 1–10.

[40] Spitzer WO, Skovron ML, Salmi LR, et al. Scientific monograph of the Quebec Task Force on whiplash-associated disorders: redefining "whiplash" and its management. Spine 1995; 20:1S–73S.

[41] Rodriquez AA, Barr KP, Burns SP. Whiplash: pathophysiology, diagnosis, treatment, and prognosis. Muscle Nerve 2004;29:768–81.

[42] Ovadia D, Steinberg EL, Nissan M, et al. Whiplash injury: a retrospective study on patients seeking compensation. Injury 2002;33:569–73.

[43] Ronnen HR, de Korte PJ, Brink PR, et al. Acute whiplash injury: is there a role for MR imaging? A prospective study of 100 patients. Radiology 1996;201:93–6.

[44] Borchgrevink G, Smevik O, Haave I, et al. MRI of the cerebrum and cervical column within two days after whiplash neck sprain injury. Injury 1997;28:331–5.

[45] Pettersson K, Hildingsson C, Toolanen G, et al. Disc pathology after whiplash injury: a prospective magnetic resonance imaging and clinical investigation. Spine 1997;22:283–7.

[46] Jonsson H, Cesarini K, Sahlstedt B, et al. Findings and outcome in whiplash-type neck distortions. Spine 1994;19:2733–43.

[47] Cothren CC, Moore EE, Biffl WL, et al. Anticoagulation is the gold standard therapy for blunt carotid injuries to reduce stroke rate. Arch Surg 2004;139:540–5 [discussion: 545–6].

[48] Cothren CC, Moore EE, Biffl WL, et al. Cervical spine fracture patterns predictive of blunt vertebral artery injury. J Trauma 2003;55:811–3.

[49] Biffl WL, Moore EE, Offner PJ, et al. Blunt carotid and vertebral arterial injuries. World J Surg 2001; 25:1036–43.

[50] Biffl WL, Moore EE, Elliott JP, et al. The devastating potential of blunt vertebral arterial injuries. Ann Surg 2000;231:672–81.

[51] Gaskill-Shipley MF, Tomsick TA. Angiography in the evaluation of head and neck trauma. Neuroimaging Clin N Am 1996;6:607–24.

[52] Shah GV, Quint DJ, Trobe JD. Magnetic resonance imaging of suspected cervicocranial arterial dissections. J Neuroophthalmol 2004;24: 315–8.

[53] Ofer A, Nitecki SS, Braun J, et al. CT angiography of the carotid arteries in trauma to the neck. Eur J Vasc Endovasc Surg 2001;21:401–7.

[54] Munera F, Soto JA, Nunez D. Penetrating injuries of the neck and the increasing role of CTA. Emerg Radiol 2004;10(6):303–9.

[55] Hollingworth W, Nathens AB, Kanne JP, et al. The diagnostic accuracy of computed tomography angiography for traumatic or atherosclerotic lesions of the carotid and vertebral arteries: a systematic review. Eur J Radiol 2003; 48:88–102.

[56] Silberstein M, Tress BM, Hennessy O. Delayed neurologic deterioration in the patient with spinal trauma: role of MR imaging. AJNR Am J Neuroradiol 1992;13:1373–81.

ELSEVIER
SAUNDERS

RADIOLOGIC
CLINICS
OF NORTH AMERICA

Radiol Clin N Am 44 (2006) 13–39

Imaging of Traumatic Neurovascular Injury

M.J.B. Stallmeyer, MD, PhD[a],*, Robert E. Morales, MD[a],
Adam E. Flanders, MD[b]

- The spectrum of vascular injury
- Clinical presentation
- Imaging
- Specific problems in neurovascular traumatic injury
  Vascular injuries of the neck resulting from penetrating trauma
  Blunt traumatic cervicocerebral vascular injury

  Extracranial head and neck arteriovenous fistulas
  Facial trauma and epistaxis
  Intracranial dissections, aneurysms, pseudoaneurysms, and lacerations
  Intracranial arteriovenous fistula
- Summary
- References

Imaging evaluation of patients with suspected neurovascular injury can be one of the most challenging problems faced by radiologists in an emergency room or trauma center. Although traumatic cervical and cerebral vascular injuries, such as dissections, lacerations, pseudoaneurysms, occlusions, and arteriovenous fistulas (AVF), are relatively uncommon events, they can result in potentially devastating strokes. Many recent studies have demonstrated that early imaging diagnosis of neurovascular injuries, particularly those caused by blunt trauma, can help improve patient outcome by facilitating more prompt treatment of these lesions [1–4].

Traditionally, patients with suspected injury to vessels in the head and neck have been evaluated with four-vessel cervical and cerebral angiography. Although conventional digital subtraction angiography remains the current diagnostic gold standard examination [5–7], it is costly and often impractical

as a screening modality, and carries a small but finite risk of serious complication, such as stroke, acute renal failure, or death [8,9]. MR imaging and MR angiography, although quite sensitive in demonstrating cervical and intracranial vascular injury [10–14], may be difficult to obtain in unstable acutely injured patients. With recent advances in multidetector CT technology, CT angiography (CTA) has emerged as a promising technique for rapid screening evaluation of neurovascular injury [15–19], although its use in definitive diagnosis remains controversial. The best imaging pathway in any individual patient may vary with the acuity of injury; the presence of concomitant orthopedic or visceral injuries; and the therapeutic options (eg, medical, surgical, or endovascular) available in the treating institution.

This article presents a general approach to the patient with suspected neurovascular injury. Fol-

[a] Division of Diagnostic and Interventional Neuroradiology, Department of Diagnostic Radiology, University of Maryland School of Medicine, Baltimore, MD, USA
[b] Division of Neuroradiology/ENT, Department of Radiology, Thomas Jefferson University Hospital, Philadelphia, PA, USA
* Corresponding author. Division of Diagnostic and Interventional Neuroradiology, Department of Diagnostic Radiology, University of Maryland School of Medicine, 22 South Greene Street, Baltimore, MD 21208.
E-mail address: bstallmeyer@umm.edu (M.J.B. Stallmeyer).

doi:10.1016/j.rcl.2005.08.003

lowing a brief discussion of the histopathologic spectrum of arterial injury, topics addressed include clinical presentation; principles of radiologic work-up including cross-sectional modalities and angiography; mechanisms of injury; and management considerations in the most commonly seen types of vascular injury, including endovascular techniques used to treat these patients.

The spectrum of vascular injury

Although blood vessels can be injured by a variety of mechanisms, all traumatic injuries involve either partial or complete disruption of the vessel wall. Neurovascular injury can be thought of as a continuous spectrum of disease: injury ranges from minimal separation of the intima from the underlying media, through development of a dissection flap and false lumen, to medial or adventitial perforation with pseudoaneurysm formation, or, more seriously, to complete transection or occlusion. AVFs occur in the specific case where transection of an adjacent artery and vein result in communication between the two vessel lumens.

Dissection, regardless of whether it is produced by blunt or penetrating trauma, separates the layers of the arterial wall. Most commonly, the intimal layer is disrupted, resulting in formation of a false lumen as blood tracks into the subintimal space. Hemorrhage may be confined to the subintimal layer, or may extend through the media or adventitia. Blood tracking along the subintimal space tends to produce luminal narrowing. In contrast, blood extending into the subadventitial space tends to weaken the vessel, and can result in apparent luminal widening as a pseudoaneurysm forms. In either case, an enlarging false lumen or pseudoaneurysm can further compromise flow through the true lumen, with progression to vessel occlusion. Occlusions are more common in patients with penetrating injury [20].

When dissection occurs, thrombus may form on the injured intimal lining, or may occur as a result of static flow within a pseudoaneurysm, false lumen, or markedly narrowed true lumen. Distal thromboembolism occurs in a significant proportion of patients with traumatic cervical carotid or vertebral arterial dissections and pseudoaneurysms, with consequent risk of stroke and death [2,5,17,20–31]. Stroke resulting from hemodynamic compromise as a result of cervical arterial occlusion alone is less common [32].

The most severe degree of injury is complete transection of the vessel. Many patients with transection of a large artery, such as the internal carotid or vertebral, exsanguinate before reaching medical attention, and those who survive to reach hospital have a high risk of stroke or death despite aggressive surgical or endovascular management [21,33–35].

Clinical presentation

Patients with neurovascular injury typically present to the emergency department with one or more of the following: an acute neurologic deficit; a history of blunt force or penetrating trauma (acute, subacute, or remote); or obvious signs of trauma by visual inspection.

Patients with carotid dissection most commonly complain of pain in the neck, face, scalp, or head ipsilateral to the side of dissection [36]. Pain, which is seen as the sole presenting symptom in 15% of patients, may be mild or severe, but more often is dull and nonthrobbing. Other presenting symptoms include pulsatile tinnitus; asymptomatic bruit; Horner syndrome (40%); and cranial neuropathies [37,38]. Vertebral artery dissections most commonly present with posterior unilateral headache with or without neck pain.

Stroke or transient ischemic attack is the next most common initial presenting symptom in both carotid and vertebral dissections. Neurologic symptoms secondary to traumatic vascular injury may be immediate or delayed [2,24,29,30,39,40], sometimes lagging behind appearance of other symptoms, such as pain or headache, by several days. About half of patients eventually developing a symptomatic dissection have a normal neurologic examination at presentation [26].

External signs suggestive of possible extracranial or intracranial neurovascular arterial injury include penetrating wound to the neck, face, or orbit; epistaxis; hemorrhage from the mouth, orbit, or ears; periorbital ecchymosis or Battle's sign; expanding cervical hematoma or pulsatile mass; cervical bruising or abrasions; and cervical bruit in a young patient.

Imaging

Both CT and MR imaging cross-sectional methods have a role in imaging of traumatic neurovascular injury. CT is the imaging modality of choice for the initial evaluation of patients with traumatic head injury and patients who develop an acute change in neurologic status following trauma. With the increased speed of image acquisition and improved resolution available in newer multidetector scanners, CT imaging is increasingly replacing plain X-ray films in the initial evaluation of neck and cervical spine trauma. In most medical centers treating trauma patients, CT can be obtained quickly and easily 24 hours a day, and is preferred in the acute stages of care [41]. Although MR imaging is the most sensitive test for evaluating the extent of brain injury [42,43], it has no significant advantage over CT in the evaluation of acute patients [44]. In the severely injured acute trauma patient, availability of 24-hour radiology technologist support and the need for specialized ventilators, intravenous pumps, and monitoring equipment may curtail practical use of this modality. Transport factors also play a role, because in many institutions the MR imaging scanner is located some distance from the emergency room or trauma unit.

Noncontrast CT has long been a standard examination for assessment of penetrating and blunt neck injuries, which not uncommonly are associated with neurovascular injury. Signs suspicious for vascular injury on noncontrast CT include prevertebral soft tissue swelling, hematoma adjacent to a large vessel or along the trajectory of the penetrating object, infiltration of perivascular fat planes, and bone and bullet fragments less than 5 mm from a major vessel [15,45]. Types of fracture predisposing to neurovascular injury include atlantoaxial dissociation; hangman's fracture; and cervical spine vertebral body fracture-dislocations, especially perched or jumped facet dislocations and C2-C6 foramen transversarium fractures [39,46–51].

At the authors' institution, MR imaging of the neck and cervical spine is most typically performed in trauma patients in whom there is concern for spinal cord injury, ligamentous disruption, traumatic disk herniation, or hemorrhage within the spinal canal. As is the case for CT, certain types of fracture and abnormal signal within perivascular soft tissues or the foramen transversarium are clues suggesting that neurovascular injury may be present. Additionally, cross-sectional MR imaging may reveal the false lumen of a dissection as a crescent of T1-hyperintense clot along the periphery of the arterial wall, or occlusion of the vessel as T1-hyperintense signal within the lumen.

Patients with suspected intracranial injury are initially evaluated with noncontrast head CT to evaluate for intracranial hemorrhage. In the setting of penetrating trauma or significant blunt injury to the head, the presence of parenchymal hematoma, subarachnoid hemorrhage, or intraventricular blood may herald the presence of an intracranial traumatic aneurysm, pseudoaneurysm, or dissecting aneurysm. Types of skull fracture raising a question of traumatic neurovascular injury include displaced midface fractures [39,52] and basilar skull fractures, especially those that extend through the petrous carotid canal or the region of the cavernous sinus [39,53–55]. These findings, however, are not highly specific for neurovascular injury [46].

MR imaging is superior to noncontrast CT in detecting early signs of intracranial ischemia secondary to vascular pathology [56,57], but because of the logistics and time costs of transporting trauma patients to the MR imager, it is seldom used in the acute setting. It is, however, the method of choice in detecting diffuse axonal injury [58], which suggests the patient has experienced significant deceleration forces [59] and is at risk for intracranial neurovascular injury.

The major shortcoming of noncontrast CT in evaluation of cervical and cerebral vascular trauma is that the presence of injury is inferred from the indirect findings described previously. Although MR imaging may accurately demonstrate subintimal thrombus in dissection, it is difficult to differentiate slow-flow lesions from occlusions. CTA and MR angiography are better at demonstrating direct signs of vascular injury, such as irregular margins of the vessel, filling defects within the contrast column, caliber changes of the vessel, extravasation of contrast, and vascular occlusion [18,60–62].

With recent advances in multidetector CT technology, it has become possible to perform rapid CTA evaluation of patients with suspected traumatic neurovascular injury in a matter of minutes [Table 1] [16,18,19,63,64]. Although digital subtraction angiography is still considered the gold standard for evaluating the cervical and cerebral vasculature, CTA is less invasive; less resource-intensive; and has the added benefit of simultaneously visualizing extravascular structures, such as the airway, brain, and spinal canal. These features make CTA an attractive alternative to catheter angiography. In at least some cases, CTA can provide sufficient information to alter triage decisions in the acute trauma patient. For example, a patient with obvious vascular injury on CTA can proceed immediately to definitive surgical or endovascular intervention. Conversely, a

Table 1: Sample CTA protocol for evaluation of cervical and intracerebral vessels for potential traumatic neurovascular injury

Parameter	Carotid CTA
kVp	120
mAs/Slice	245
FOV	220
Thickness (mm)	1
Increment (mm)	0.5
Rotation time (sec)	.75
Collimation	16 × 0.75
Pitch	0.9
Injection	100 mL at 4 mL/s
Trigger	120 HU at the ascending aorta
Scan	Inferior to superior from the aortic arch to 1 cm above the Circle of Willis

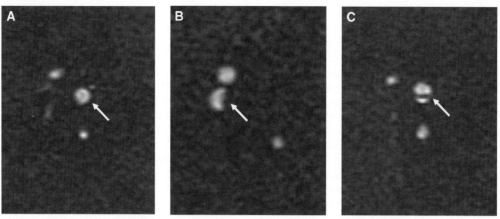

Fig. 1. MR angiography appearance of dissection. Axial source images from two-dimensional time-of-flight MR angiography sequence demonstrate (*arrows*) (*A*) the round contour of flow signal within a normal cervical right internal carotid artery (ICA), (*B*) flattening of the medial margin of the flow signal caused by a thrombosed false lumen within a dissected right ICA, and (*C*) flow signal within both the true and false lumens, separated by an intraluminal flap, within a dissected right ICA.

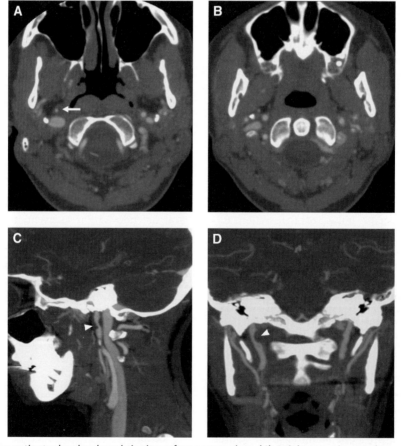

Fig. 2. CTA of a patient who developed tinnitus after a yoga class. (*A*) Axial source image demonstrates round contour, but decreased caliber of a dissected right ICA at the level of a nearly concentric false lumen (*arrow*). Compare with (*B*) an axial source image from slightly more caudad in the neck where the ICAs are virtually identical in caliber. Sagittal (*C*) and coronal planar (*D*) reconstructions demonstrate the nonopacifying false lumen in the dissected right ICA (*arrowheads*) and minimal irregularity in the left ICA, which was seen at angiography to be normal.

patient with low suspicion for injury and a normal CTA may have their angiographic procedure timed more appropriately with respect to management of concomitant limb or visceral injuries, or may be able to forego the risk of conventional angiography entirely. Later in the trauma patient's clinical course, either CTA or MR angiography may be helpful in evaluating interval healing of injury.

The same basic principles are used in interpreting CT and MR angiographic images in the setting of trauma. The hallmark of vascular injury is a change in the caliber of the vessel. A normal artery maintains a nearly constant diameter between branch points and, with the notable exception of the carotid bulb, an artery does not increase in caliber as it courses from proximal to distal. Because the common carotid arteries, internal carotid arteries (ICA), and vertebral arteries travel for long distances within the neck without giving off major branches, any notable change in caliber should raise concern for injury. A normal artery also maintains a consistently rounded cross-section, except on turns. On CTA, an oval, irregular, or slit-like cross-section may indicate the presence of a dissection flap with a nonopacifying false lumen. On MR angiography, the equivalent finding may indicate either a lack of flow signal within the false lumen or extramural hematoma compressing the vessel [**Fig. 1A**]. If the false lumen opacifies with contrast on CTA, or contains flow signal or T1-hyperintense methemoglobin clot on MR angiography, the dissection flap may appear as a linear filling defect within the contrast column [**Fig. 1C**]. When the vascular injury presents as a subtle change in caliber, but maintains a rounded shape, minimal intimal injury or a small dissection is suspected [**Fig. 2**].

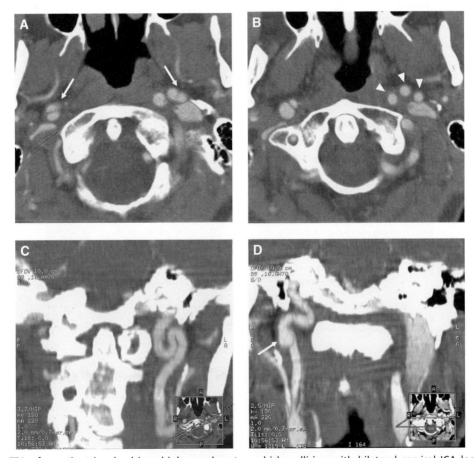

Fig. 3. CTA of a patient involved in a high-speed motor vehicle collision with bilateral cervical ICA loops and dissection of the right ICA. (*A*) Axial source image demonstrates what seem to be bilateral ICA dissections, with contrast within true and false lumens separated by an intraluminal flap (*arrows*). (*B*) An axial source image from slightly more caudad in the neck, however, demonstrates three clearly separated round ICA lumens on the left (*arrowheads*), consistent with a vascular loop. Oblique coronal planar reconstructed images clearly demonstrate (*C*) the loop in the uninjured left ICA and (*D*) a pseudoaneurysm in the distal cervical right ICA (*arrow*), which also has a loop in its course. The split in contrast columns on source images is seen to correspond to a dissection flap and pseudoaneurysm in the right ICA, whereas on the left it identifies the apex of the turn in the loop.

A multitude of planar and three-dimensional reconstructed views can be generated from the axial CTA and MR angiography source images; these allow the vessel to be studied from any angle. Both the axial source images and reconstructed images are evaluated for the presence of injury. In interpreting axial images, it is essential to follow the course of each vessel, not only for its complete interrogation, but to avoid misnaming a vessel or misinterpreting a vascular loop as a pseudoaneurysm. For example, in evaluating the cervical ICA, the artery is followed on source images in stack mode from its origin to the petrous carotid canal at the skull base. This is particularly important when the ICA is in close proximity to the internal jugular vein or external carotid branches, because these are often not easily separated on the reconstructed

images. This technique is also important when the carotid or vertebral arteries are redundant or looped, to differentiate turns in the vessel from a pseudoaneurysm. In most cases, scrolling back and forth in the axial source images as the vessel turns back caudally reveals the correct diagnosis, which should then be confirmed on the reconstructed images [Fig. 3].

Evaluation of the reconstructed images is performed essentially in the same manner as interpreting conventional angiographic images. In more severe injury grades (eg, large pseudoaneurysms, occlusions, or lacerations with contrast extravasation), findings are obvious on both the source and reconstructed image sets. In milder degrees of injury, the information they provide is often complimentary. In general, deviations from a round

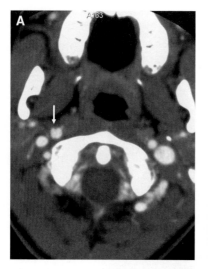
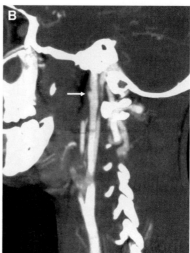
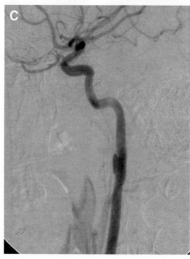

Fig. 4. CTA of a patient involved in a motor vehicle collision. Axial source image (*A*) and sagittal planar reconstruction (*B*) demonstrate a small pseudoaneurysm in the distal cervical right ICA (*arrows*). (C) Digital subtraction angiography (DSA) of the right ICA in lateral projection confirms the diagnosis.

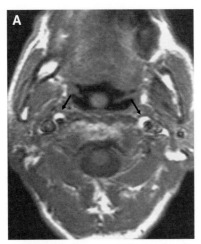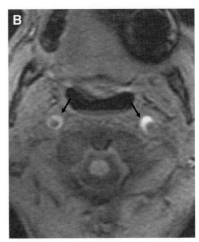

Fig. 5. Axial T1-weighted MR images, without (*A*) and with (*B*) fat-saturation technique, demonstrate high signal methemoglobin clot within the false lumens of bilateral ICA dissections (*arrows*). This can often be detected more easily on fat-saturated images.

cross-section are more easily detected on the axial images, whereas changes in caliber are often more obvious on the reconstructed images. The true extent and nature of the lesion is usually more easily perceived on the reconstructed images. To some degree, this is likely a consequence of the similarity in appearance of reconstructed images to conventional angiographic images; however, the craniocaudal extent of an injury is often not intuitively perceived on axial images, but is readily visible on reconstructions. Reconciling findings between the two sets of images usually confirms the diagnosis [Fig. 4].

Cross-sectional MR imaging may have a slight advantage in detection of milder degrees of injury, where the only finding may be subtle uplifting of the endothelium by a small subintimal hematoma.

Axial T1-weighted MR imaging may demonstrate a thin crescent of methemoglobin clot in the false lumen along the periphery of the arterial wall. Applying fat saturation technique to suppress the high signal in the surrounding abundant fat throughout the neck increases the sensitivity in detecting this finding [Figs. 5 and 6].

Pseudoaneurysms can have a variable appearance, depending on whether blood or contrast flows into the pseudoaneurysm sac, or whether the sac is filled by thrombus. On both CTA and MR angiography, a patent pseudoaneurysm sac has the appearance of a focal outpouching from the artery of origin. On CTA a thrombosed pseudoaneurysm or thrombosed false lumen appears as an eccentric and usually smooth filling defect in or adjacent to the true lumen [Fig. 7]. On MR imaging,

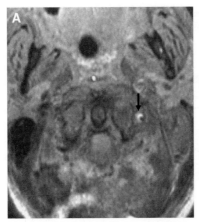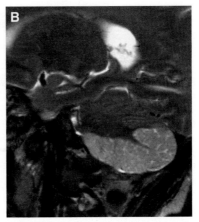

Fig. 6. Dissection with thromboembolism and infarct. (*A*) Axial fat-saturated T1-weighted MR image demonstrates methemoglobin within the false lumen (*arrow*) of a left vertebral artery dissection. (*B*) Sagittal T2-weighted MR image depicts a large posterior inferior cerebellar artery infarct.

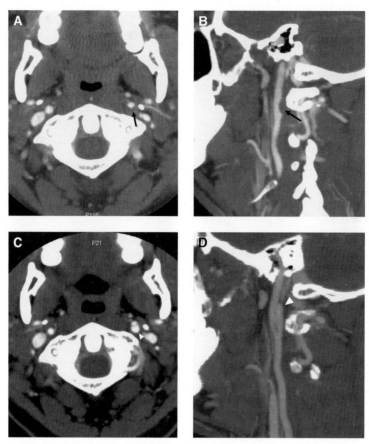

Fig. 7. CTA of a patient with C5 and C6 fractures following a motor vehicle accident, with an enlarging left ICA pseudoaneurysm. Axial source (*A*) and sagittal planar reformatted (*B*) images at the time of admission demonstrate a small eccentric dissection with nonopacifying false lumen along the posterior aspect of the left ICA (*arrows*), for which he received anticoagulation therapy. Three months later, follow-up axial source image (*C*) and sagittal planar reconstruction (*D*) demonstrate a large pseudoaneurysm (*arrowhead*) at the same site.

the appearance depends on the age of any formed thrombus; large pseudoaneurysms and older thrombosed pseudoaneurysms often have a heterogeneous, complex signal pattern [Fig. 8].

AVFs present a number of difficulties in diagnosis on CTA and MR angiography, because the hallmark of this type of injury is early filling of a vein. Although this finding can be demonstrated with CT perfusion images [65], at the present state of technology the anatomic details of the fistulous connection are not particularly well delineated on most scanners. Furthermore, reliable timing of the contrast bolus so that early filling of a vein in arterial phase is detected can be difficult; simply seeing unilateral contrast opacification of the cavernous sinus on CTA is not a specific finding for carotid-cavernous fistula (CCF). Time-resolved MR angiography [66] may prove to be amenable to demonstrating these lesions directly but is not widely available. The definitive diagnosis of a cervical AVF or CCF is made on conventional angiography. If, however, there is

sufficient pressure transfer through the fistula, dilatation of cervical veins, the superior ophthalmic vein, and dural venous sinuses may provide indirect evidence for the presence of an AVF [Fig. 9]. In CCF, venous congestion of the extraocular muscles and orbital fat can also contribute to the diagnosis [Fig. 10].

Despite the encouraging results reported in multiple studies in which CTA has been used to evaluate patients with possible neurovascular injury [16,18, 19,63,64], there are still some disadvantages inherent in this modality. Bullet fragments, other metallic penetrating objects, and dental amalgams can result in streak artifact that obscures portions of the vessels. Blood vessels surrounded by bone, such as the ICA as it penetrates the skull base or the vertebral artery as it courses through the foramen transversarium, can be difficult to visualize and evaluate in their entirety [63]. At the current state of technology, the total contrast load administered to the patient typically exceeds that given in digital sub-

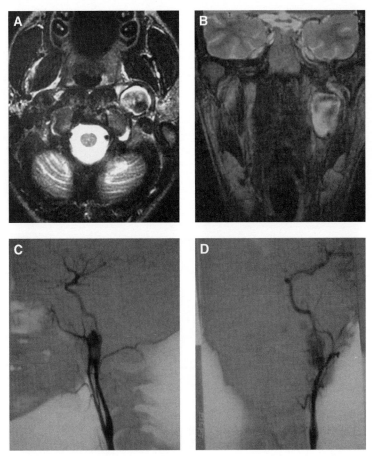

Fig. 8. Heterogeneous MR imaging signal in large pseudoaneurysm. Axial (*A*) and coronal (*B*) T2-weighted images demonstrate a large pseudoaneurysm adjacent to the left ICA with a complex signal pattern. This can represent areas of thrombus adjacent to a patent lumen, or slow disordered flow within the pseudoaneurysm sac. Lateral (*C*) and anteroposterior (*D*) DSA of the left common carotid demonstrates filling of most of the pseudoaneurysm sac, with irregular thrombus along its medial border.

traction angiography. Furthermore, it can sometimes be difficult to time the contrast bolus so that all structures of interest are imaged exclusively during arterial phase. For example, opacification of venous structures abutting an artery may obscure a crucial finding or be mistaken for an arterial abnormality, and early venous filling in an AVF cannot always be reliably seen. Overall, however, the percentage of nondiagnostic studies has been reported to be low at approximately 1% [18], and even in instances where all major vessels cannot be cleared by CTA, the identification of clearly normal, uninjured vessels can focus the scope of a subsequent angiographic study.

Patients referred for angiographic evaluation or for endovascular treatment of cervicocerebral vascular injury or severe facial bleeding and epistaxis following trauma often have multiple injuries, and may be hemodynamically unstable. Appropriate triage to ensure that the most life-threatening inju-

ries (whether visceral, limb, or craniofacial) are treated first is crucial; careful review of all available CT imaging, and discussion of clinical findings with the referring emergency room or trauma physician, should be performed to identify all potential sources of bleeding.

Intubation or tracheostomy to protect the airway is mandatory in severely injured patients undergoing angiography. Even in a cooperative and conscious patient, prophylactic intubation before angiography is often prudent if a decline in level of consciousness is anticipated, or if the patient presented with bleeding, which could potentially compromise the airway should hemorrhage recur during the procedure. Some patients may have had packing placed in the oropharynx or nasopharynx to control hemorrhage; this may obscure the site of bleeding but should probably be left in place unless the origin of bleeding cannot be identified or inferred from angiographic findings.

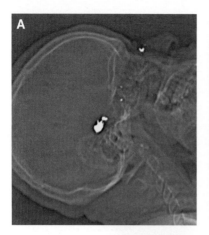
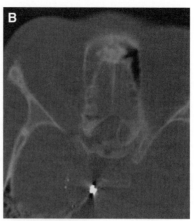
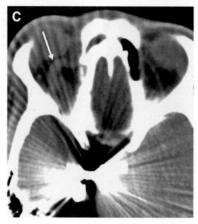

Fig. 9. CCF secondary to gunshot wound. Scout (*A*) and axial (*B*) CT images depicted in bone windows demonstrate a bullet trajectory, with a large ballistic fragment adjacent to the right cavernous sinus. (*C*) Axial CT image in soft tissue window demonstrates enlargement of the ipsilateral superior ophthalmic vein (*arrow*), a finding suspicious for CCF.

Arch aortography is often a useful first step to evaluate for thoracic and cervical great vessel injury. Attention can then be given to evaluate for large cervical vessel injury, and finally for intracranial injury. The role of careful angiographic technique cannot be overemphasized. A suspected site of injury should not be crossed with the catheter or wire until angiography or road mapping has demonstrated that passage can be performed with a reasonable degree of safety, because inadvertent further injury to the artery or dislodgement of intraluminal thrombus may occur.

A detailed discussion of the issues in endovascular therapy of traumatic neurovascular injury is beyond the scope of this article, but brief summaries of options appropriate to various types of injury are described next. As a general principle, however, before any endovascular embolization or stenting procedure, a baseline cerebral angiogram should be obtained; this should be repeated at the end of the procedure to evaluate for any intracranial arterial embolization that may have occurred.

Specific problems in neurovascular traumatic injury

Vascular injuries of the neck resulting from penetrating trauma

Approximately 25% of patients with penetrating neck trauma have vascular injury [25,35,67–70]. Many penetrating vascular injuries result from direct violation of the vessel wall by a bullet or sharp object. Gunshot wounds, however, may sometimes cause injury to blood vessels outside the zone of the bullet channel; as the projectile loses velocity and energy in tissue, the resultant shock wave produces a transient cavity in the region surrounding the bullet track, which can disrupt blood vessels [71]. In either case, assessment of trajectory is an important con-

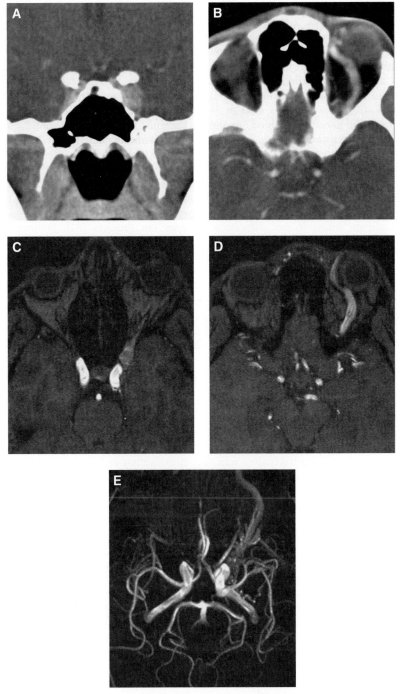

Fig. 10. CCF secondary to blunt trauma. Coronal (*A*) and axial (*B*) CTA images demonstrate enlargement of left cavernous sinus and dilatation of the left superior ophthalmic vein and asymmetric vascular congestion in the posterior left orbit. MR angiography source images (*C* and *D*) and maximum intensity projection (MIP) reconstructions (*E*) confirm arterial flow in the left cavernous sinus and left superior ophthalmic vein.

sideration in determining whether vascular injury may be present and in choosing modalities for imaging work-up.

Penetrating wounds to the carotid artery are classified by their position with respect to anatomic landmarks: (1) zone I injuries, located between the sternal notch and cricoid cartilage; (2) zone II injuries, between the cricoid cartilage and the angle of the mandible; and (3) zone III injuries, between the angle of the mandible and the skull base.

Because direct surgical exploration of zone I or III carotid injuries may be difficult, considerable premium is placed on preoperative imaging assessment to locate the exact site of vascular injury. In contrast, patients with zone II carotid injuries, particularly if blood loss is clinically obvious, may be explored surgically without prior imaging.

Vertebral artery injury may occur as a result of direct trauma from the penetrating object, or the penetrating object may fracture a cervical vertebra, secondarily causing injury to the artery as it courses through the foramen transversarium or stretches around splintered or displaced bones. This latter mechanism is particularly prevalent in gunshot wounds [72].

Penetrating traumatic injury to the extracranial carotid or vertebral arteries carries significant risk of stroke [20,21,73]. Whenever the patient's neurologic deficit is not explained adequately by head CT findings, major cervical vascular injury should be considered. Because early ischemic changes may not be apparent on noncontrast CT [74], patients presenting with neurovascular territorial symptoms after head or neck injury may require emergent evaluation with CTA and CT perfusion, which increases sensitivity for detection of early infarcts [75], or conventional angiography.

Noncontrast and contrast CT are usually the best modalities for initial assessment of penetrating vascular injury in the neck. Although predicting the course of bullet fragments or other penetrating metal objects at the time of the initial trauma is not completely reliable, often a better understanding of the trajectory can be obtained with CT imaging than on plain films, or even from physical examination. The location of the entrance wound, air droplets, disrupted structures, infiltrated fat planes, focal hematomas, and final location of projectile fragments aid in predicting the course of penetrating objects. Until the location of all metal fragments is determined, MR imaging is at least relatively contraindicated because of the dangers of fragment migration or heating effects [76,77]. Close proximity of blood vessels to the path of fragments, or to the zone of damage caused by a ballistic shock wave, increases the probability of neurovascular injury. Visualizing injuries to other major structures, including the airway, alimentary tract, and spine, is also essential in the triage of these patients for future management decisions. Patients with zone I or III penetrating carotid vascular injury usually require conventional angiography in addition to CT, and may require endovascular management. Patients with zone II carotid injury can often be assessed with CT or CTA [15,18, 78,79], but may also require conventional angiography. If the penetrating object has caused cervical spine fracture, there is a significant risk of vertebral artery injury, which in many cases requires conventional angiography and possibly endovascular therapy.

When milder degrees of penetrating neurovascular injury, such as minimal intimal injury and nonhemodynamically significant dissection flaps, are present, the goal of treatment is primarily to prevent distal thromboembolism and stroke. Systemic anticoagulation with heparin and warfarin has been shown to be effective in "spontaneous" dissections and those caused by blunt injury [26,80,81], and is probably effective in less serious penetrating dissections as well, as long as it is not contraindicated by other injuries and the dissection does not progress [82]. Preliminary results with treatment with antiplatelet agents is promising [83], but no randomized trials comparing anticoagulation with antiplatelet agents in treatment of dissection have been performed [84].

Treatment of more severe degrees of injury, such as pseudoaneurysm or arterial laceration, depends largely on the location of the lesion. Zone II carotid injuries are often treated surgically with primary repair or an interposition graft [82]. In zones I and III carotid injury, endovascular repair may be preferred. Various endovascular repair techniques used include coil embolization of the vessel stump in arterial occlusions, reconstruction of a partially patent artery with self-expanding or balloon-expandable stents, primary coiling of pseudoaneurysms, or stent and coil embolization of pseudoaneurysms [33,85–87], with trapping of the pseudoaneurysm with vessel sacrifice used as a last resort [Fig. 11]. Recent reports have described success in using covered stent-grafts in closing lacerations and pseudoaneurysms of the extracranial ICA caused by penetrating injury [85,88–91]. Lacerated vertebral arteries are often difficult to approach surgically, and are usually treated by endovascular occlusion of the artery [92–94]. Unilateral vertebral artery occlusion seldom results in neurologic deficits if the contralateral vertebral artery is not injured, is of adequate size, and the posteroinferior cerebellar artery blood supply on the side of occlusion is preserved.

Blunt traumatic cervicocerebral vascular injury

Neurovascular injury caused by blunt force mechanisms is a relatively uncommon but potentially devastating event. Centers performing aggressive screening for blunt force vascular injury have reported an incidence of carotid injury of 0.33% to 3.5%, depending on mechanism [3,4,16,17,95], and an incidence of vertebral injury of 0.53% to 0.71% [2,17]. The mortality rate from posttraumatic extracranial carotid dissection ranges, however, from 20% to 40% in reported series, and

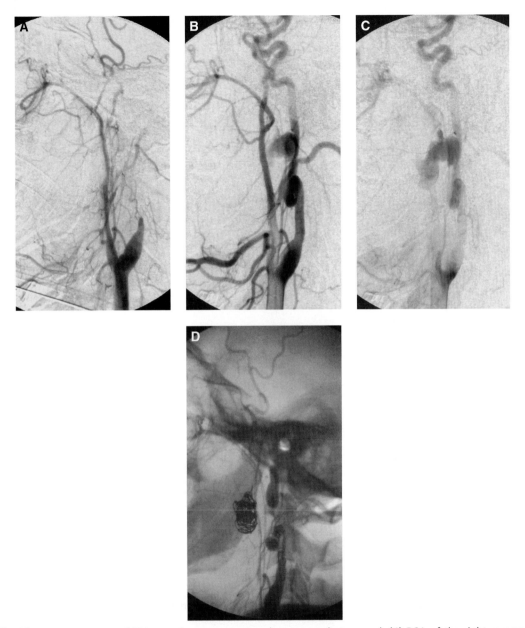

Fig. 11. Late appearance of ICA pseudoaneurysm secondary to gunshot wound. (*A*) DSA of the right common carotid at the time of admission demonstrates occlusion of the right ICA. Four days later, the patient developed increased swelling near the mandibular angle. Repeat DSA in early (*B*) and late (*C*) arterial phase demonstrates a large, slowly filling pseudoaneurysm near the skull base. The previously noted occlusion was thought to be secondary to spasm. Endovascular occlusion of the wide-necked pseudoaneurysm was attempted, but a prominent loop in the mid-ICA proximal to the pseudoaneurysm precluded passage of a stent across the pseudoaneurysm neck. (*D*) Following successful balloon test occlusion of the right ICA without development of neurologic deficit, the pseudoaneurysm was trapped and the artery was sacrificed using a combination of detachable balloons and coils.

significant neurologic sequelae have been reported to occur in between 12.5% and 80% of survivors [2,5,17,20,22,23,26–31]. The corresponding mortality and neurologic morbidity rates for extracranial vertebral artery injury are 4% to 8% and 14% to 24%, respectively [2,24]. Cervicocerebral arterial dissection, including spontaneous dissections and those occurring after minor trauma, is estimated to cause about 1% of all ischemic strokes, and 5% of ischemic strokes in young adults [96,97].

Mechanisms producing high risk of blunt carotid and vertebral injury include direct blows to the neck, and deceleration injuries producing high shearing forces from a stretching or twisting motion of the neck [5,24,98]. Basilar skull fractures that cross the petrous carotid canal can also produce carotid injury at this level [46]. Motor vehicle collisions, falls, and assaults are the most common mechanisms [2,28,40]. Additional etiologies of blunt injury to the extracranial carotid and vertebral artery include chiropractic manipulation [99–103], sports activity [104–109], and rapid head turning or flexion-extension movements [110,111].

In blunt trauma, cross-sectional imaging provides fewer clues regarding the vectors of force causing injury than are present when injury results from penetrating mechanisms. By definition, culpable foreign bodies are absent, and air bubbles tracking

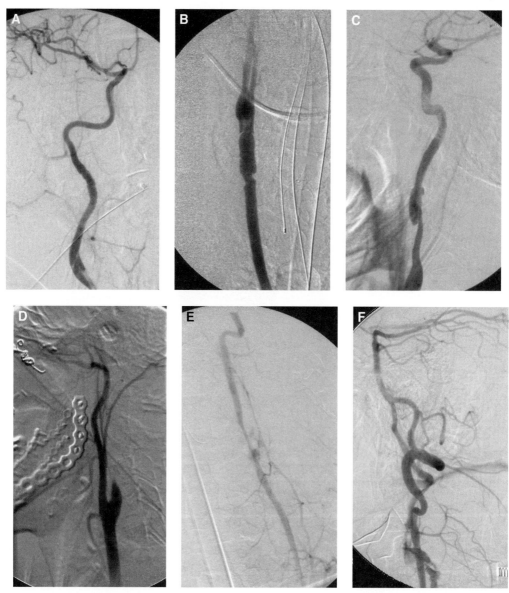

Fig. 12. Vascular injury scale of Biffl. (*A*) Grade I: the hallmark of this degree of injury is irregularity of the vessel wall. A dissection flap, with less than 25% luminal compromise, may also be present. (*B*) Grade II: dissection with greater than 25% luminal narrowing is present. Intraluminal thrombus may be present, and lesions may be near-occlusive. (*C*) Grade III: pseudoaneurysms appear as outpouchings from the vessel lumen. These occur most commonly in the distal cervical segment, just below the skull base. (*D*) Grade IV: the internal carotid artery is occluded just beyond the carotid bulb. (*E*) Grade V: transection of the left vertebral artery. (*F*) Grade V: transection of the left vertebral artery in the same patient (compare with [E] taken at different time and different oblique view). Gross extravasation of contrast is seen.

through the soft tissues may originate from the lungs or viscera remote from the area of interest. Infiltration of the fat planes can be present but is often less obvious. Often, one must assume traumatic forces were experienced throughout the entire neck. It is useful, however, to pay particular attention to the more likely areas of injury and dissection; for example, the distal cervical ICA just below the skull base and distal cervical vertebral artery are particularly prone to dissection as a result of blunt trauma. This is thought to occur as a consequence of the different deceleration and shearing forces experienced by an arterial segment constrained by bone, versus a segment constrained only by soft tissues. Similarly, there should be high suspicion for vertebral artery injury when cervical subluxation, or cervical spine fractures extending through the foramen transversarium are present, because both result in significant shearing forces.

Many patients require angiographic evaluation. Biffl and coworkers [34] [**Fig. 12**] designed a grading scale describing the spectrum of blunt carotid injury, based on the angiographic appearance of lesions, which also can be extended to describe vertebral artery injury [Box 1].

As is the case for corresponding penetrating injuries, the goal of therapy, both in the acute and ongoing setting, is to prevent stroke resulting from thromboembolic complications. Blunt carotid and vertebral artery injury carries a significant risk of neurologic injury and death. Although systemic anticoagulation with heparin and warfarin has been shown to be effective in treatment of blunt carotid and vertebral arterial injury in most grades of injury [1,3,26,28,34], many patients with blunt neurovascular injury have concomitant intracranial, visceral, or limb injuries that effectively preclude safe anticoagulation, at least in the acute phase. Even when anticoagulation or antiplatelet therapy [83] is administered later in the patient's course, careful surveillance for hemorrhagic complications is necessary. Many authors have reported success with stent and covered stent placement for treatment of dissections and pseudoaneurysms, sometimes with coil occlusion of the pseudoaneurysm sac [34,86,112–118]. Recently, however,

Cothren and coworkers [119] have raised concerns regarding complication rates and long-term patency in patients with grade III blunt carotid injuries (pseudoaneurysms) treated with stents; many patients in their series, however, did not receive long-term antiplatelet therapy as has been advocated for patients having stents placed for treatment of carotid bifurcation atherosclerosis [120], and other studies have reported good long-term patency [121].

Extracranial head and neck arteriovenous fistulas

AVF in the neck and scalp are most commonly seen as a result of penetrating trauma [122]. In the neck, high-flow fistulous connections most commonly involve the common or ICAs and internal jugular vein, or external carotid artery main trunk and internal jugular vein. High-flow AVF involving the vertebral artery and internal jugular vein or vertebral veins has also been reported [123–126]. AVF involving branches of the external carotid artery, because of smaller vessel size, demonstrates a smaller degree of shunting.

Patients most commonly present with a pulsatile neck or scalp mass, hemorrhage, bruit, or complain of tinnitus or headache. As with traumatic dissections, stroke may occur as a result of the injury [21]. Although cervical AVF may demonstrate an impressive arterial steal phenomenon at angiography, cerebral hypoperfusion or heart failure as a result of a cervical or scalp traumatic AVF is rare [126,127].

CT may demonstrate hematoma, pseudoaneurysm, and enlargement of the draining vein and some of its tributaries. Conventional angiography demonstrates early contrast opacification of the draining vein and often shows arterial steal distal to the fistula. The latter findings may be seen on CTA as asymmetric enhancement on the venous side of the fistula, perhaps with a subtle decrease in caliber or contrast density in the feeding artery distal to the fistula; however, this may not be reliably demonstrated on CTA. Because of the difficulty in timing the bolus strictly to the arterial phase, visualizing venous structures on CTA is typically a nonspecific finding unless contrast is not seen in other venous structures, or if there is a high suspicion for fistula and additional findings as described previously are present. As a technical note, if an underlying fistula is suspected, it may be helpful to administer contrast by the contralateral arm to avoid retrograde filling of neck veins on the side of interest generated by the force of mechanical contrast injection.

Treatment of AVF is accomplished by selectively occluding the fistula point while preserving the parent artery. This may be performed by direct

---

Box 1: Blunt carotid injury grade description

Grade I: Luminal irregularity or dissection with <25% luminal narrowing

Grade II: Dissection with >25% luminal narrowing

Grade III: Pseudoaneurysm

Grade IV: Occlusion

Grade V: Transection with free extravasation

surgical repair [128] or endovascular methods, which may include deployment of stents, covered stents, coils, or detachable balloons [**Fig. 13**] [21,125,126,129–131]. Less commonly, occlusion of the artery distal and proximal to the fistula point may be required.

Facial trauma and epistaxis

Massive maxillofacial hemorrhage may be secondary to facial or skull fractures [132–136] or penetrating trauma [137,138]. Clinical findings, such as obvious hemorrhage or expanding hematoma, may occur immediately or may be delayed.

In this setting, the role of CT evaluation for potential neurovascular injury is primarily one of determining whether active extravasation of contrast or hematoma is present, and in locating fracture planes in proximity to major vascular structures. For example, fractures of the pterygoid plates or posterior wall of the maxillary sinus in LeFort and facial smash injury can lacerate branches of the internal maxillary artery that not infrequently causes bleeding that is refractory to nasal packing. The

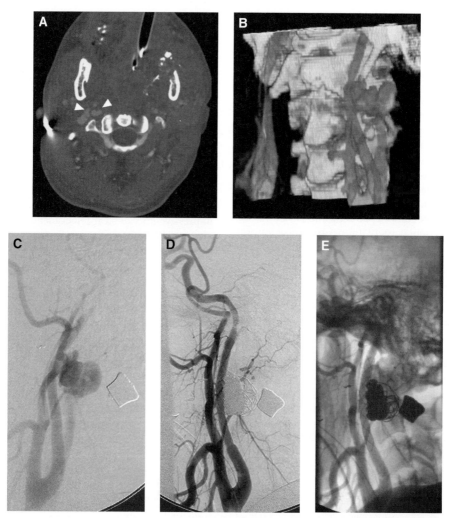

Fig. 13. Internal carotid artery to internal jugular vein fistula secondary to gunshot wound. (*A*) Axial CTA demonstrates an irregular collection of contrast adjacent to the right ICA and internal jugular vein along the bullet trajectory, which runs obliquely from right posterior to left anterior. Note left mandibular fracture. (*B*) Three-dimensional reconstructed CTA image demonstrates a large, lobulated pseudoaneurysm sac and early filling of the right internal jugular vein, with appearance identical to that seen on (*C*) lateral DSA image of the right ICA. Note lag in contrast opacification of the right ICA distal to the fistula point relative to right ECA branches, consistent with moderate steal phenomenon. The pseudoaneurysm and fistula were completely eliminated by stenting of the right ICA and coil embolization of the pseudoaneurysm sac, which communicated with the right internal jugular vein, seen in lateral DSA (*D*) and unsubtracted angiographic (*E*) images.

presence of sinus fluid in the setting of facial injury is well known to raise the question of fracture; fluid in the sphenoid sinus may be particularly alarming because this may indicate ICA injury [139,140]. Trauma to the orbits may result in retrobulbar hematoma with stretching of the optic nerve, or vascular compression and central retinal artery occlusion [141,142].

Pseudoaneurysms or transections of major branches of the external carotid artery are often best treated using coils [**Fig. 14**]. Because of the propensity of the external carotid branches to collateralize and reconstitute each other, it is important to deploy coils both distal and proximal to the injury wherever technically possible. Where smaller branches are lacerated, or where a definitive site of bleeding is not identified, the goal of treatment is to decrease the pressure head to the region of injury. In this setting, superselective embolization with polyvinyl alcohol particles in the 250- to 500-μm range is often effective. Embolization with very small particles (eg, polyvinyl alcohol < 250 μm) carries a risk of devascularization of the capillary bed and possible embolization to dangerous collaterals, such as ethmoidal branches communicating with the ophthalmic artery.

Following embolization of an injured vessel for control of facial bleeding, control angiography of both the ipsilateral and contralateral internal and external carotid arteries should be performed to evaluate potential sources of collateral supply that may cause rehemorrhage, and to rule out intracranial thromboembolic complications or inadvertent embolization of cerebral vessels by dangerous collaterals.

Intracranial dissections, aneurysms, pseudoaneurysms, and lacerations

Traumatic intracranial aneurysms and pseudoaneurysms can result from penetrating trauma, such as gunshot wounds [143–146], stab wounds [147], nail-gun injuries [148], and skull fracture with traumatic laceration or dissection of the artery [139,140]. They may also be seen in the setting of closed head injury [140,149–151], either caused by shear injury [152] or impaction of arteries against fixed dural structures, such as the falx cerebri [139,140,150]. Traumatic intracranial dissections, which may also be seen with either penetrating or blunt trauma, are encountered most frequently in the middle cerebral, vertebral, and basilar arteries [86].

Direct damage to intracranial blood vessels is potentially a life-threatening injury. Where a major brain artery is lacerated or transected, the injury is often immediately fatal, with the patient expiring from exsanguinations or the effects of elevated intracranial pressure or brain herniation [**Fig. 15**] [153]. Some cases of injury involving the supraclinoid ICA have presented with severe intractable epistaxis [86,140,154].

Traumatic intracranial aneurysms or pseudoaneurysms, particularly when caused by penetrating injury, may also appear in delayed fashion [**Fig. 16**] [155–157]. This is particularly true for high-velocity ballistic injury, where hemorrhage or thromboem-

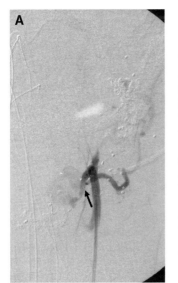 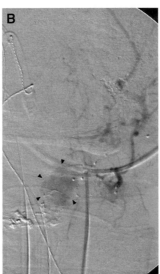 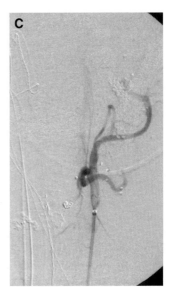

Fig. 14. Shotgun wound with laceration of the facial artery and uncontrollable hemorrhage. Oblique DSA of the left external carotid artery in arterial (*A*) and venous (*B*) phase demonstrates truncation of the left facial artery (*arrow*) with large, slowly filling pseudoaneurysm (*arrowheads*). The artery and pseudoaneurysm neck were occluded with coils (*C*).

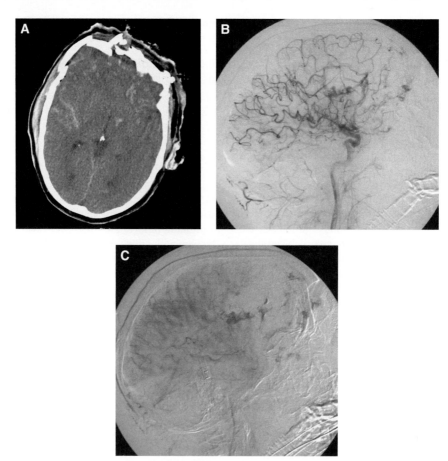

Fig. 15. Intracranial arterial lacerations and transactions with extravasation in a patient with massive skull fractures after a tree fell on his head. (*A*) CT demonstrates depressed bifrontal skull fracture, subarachnoid blood, and numerous foci of parenchymal hemorrhage. Lateral DSA of the cerebral RCCA circulation in early arterial phase (*B*) and parenchymal phase (*C*) demonstrates multiple fluffy foci of contrast extravasation in the frontal and parietal lobes. Note absent parenchymal blush and cutoff of multiple frontal branches distal to extravasation in the perisylvian region.

bolic complications may not appear until weeks or even months after the traumatic episode [143–145]. Traumatic intracranial aneurysms have a high rate of rupture, approximately 50% within the first week after injury. This type of injury should be a diagnostic consideration where initial CT evaluation demonstrates intracranial hematoma or subarachnoid blood along the trajectory of the penetrating object, or where large vessels are in proximity to the site of injury [152,158]. In one series, 3.2% of patients with subarachnoid hemorrhage following a gunshot wound to the head were found to have a traumatic intracranial aneurysm [159]. In patients with penetrating stab wounds, the incidence of traumatic intracranial aneurysm has been reported as 12% [160]. Unless the managing physician suspects the injury enough to order CTA or angiographic work-up, traumatic intracranial aneurysms and pseudoaneurysms may go undetected until a clinical disaster occurs.

Patients with suspected intracranial vascular injury likely require conventional angiography. This is particularly true for those with traumatic pseudoaneurysms, in whom endovascular treatment is likely to be considered, because in general traumatic intracranial pseudoaneurysms do not resolve spontaneously. Treatment alternatives include surgical clipping or arterial reconstruction, endovascular occlusion of the pseudoaneurysm with preservation of the parent vessel, trapping of the aneurysm by surgical or endovascular means with parent vessel sacrifice, and vascular bypass [86,161–164]. Distinguishing between true aneurysms and pseudoaneurysms on imaging is often difficult, even with cerebral angiography, because the difference between them is essentially histopathologic. In true intracranial aneurysms, the intima and adventitia are intact, whereas in intracranial pseudoaneurysms the artery is perforated and the "dome" of the pseudoaneurysm is con-

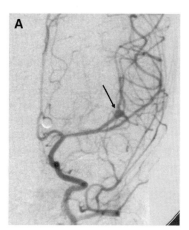 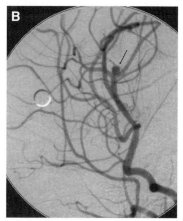

Fig. 16. Left middle cerebral artery pseudoaneurysm in a 3-month-old girl, shot with a BB with entry wound behind the ear. Seven days after admission she developed massive left basal ganglia hemorrhage. Anteroposterior (*A*) and lateral oblique (*B*) DSA of the left internal carotid circulation demonstrates a small pseudoaneurysm arising from a left middle cerebral artery posterior division branch.

tained within extraluminal clot. The lack of a defined wall in intracranial pseudoaneurysms increases the difficulty of treatment, whether by surgical or endovascular means.

Intracranial arteriovenous fistula

Intracranial AVF are most commonly seen in the setting of serious head trauma following a motor vehicle collision, assault, or penetrating injury, but also may occur after relatively minor trauma. Most posttraumatic intracranial AVF are CCF [86,165]. In these, the cavernous ICA or one of its small intracavernous branches is disrupted, resulting in a direct communication between the torn artery and the surrounding cavernous sinus. The mechanism of injury is thought to be caused by either laceration of the artery by spicules of bone associated with fracture or penetrating injury, or by tearing of the intracavernous ICA at points where it is attached to the dura, located between the foramen lacerum and the anterior clinoid process. Direct CCF may also result from rupture of a pre-existing or posttraumatic intracavernous aneurysm into the cavernous sinus. Posttraumatic direct AVF have been reported in other locations [166], but are much less common. Indirect CCF, or dural arteriovenous malformations, in which meningeal arteries communicate with venous sinuses, have also been associated with a history of trauma.

The most commonly used classification of CCF [164] divides them into four groups on the basis of arterial vascular supply [Box 2].

Barrow type-A CCF are usually high-flow fistulas and usually occur as a result of an antecedent traumatic event. In contrast, Barrow types B to D (dural arteriovenous malformations) typically dem-

onstrate relatively slow flow and occur spontaneously, although they have been associated with trauma. Analogous indirect fistulae may also occur between dural branches of the external and ICAs and other large intracerebral venous sinuses, but these seldom have a clear traumatic etiology.

The telltale angiographic finding in CCF is a nearly instantaneous filling of the ipsilateral cavernous sinus as contrast reaches the cavernous internal carotid segment. In most cases, the subcompartments of the cavernous sinus communicate freely with each other, and most commonly outflow is to the ipsilateral superior ophthalmic vein and inferior petrosal sinus. In a typical high-flow CCF, arterial-level pressure within the superior ophthalmic vein causes orbital venous hypertension, with resultant chemosis, proptosis, stretching of the optic nerve, cranial nerve deficits involving the extraocular muscles, headache, and deterioration in vision [167].

> ***Box 2:* Classification of carotid-cavernous fistulae**
>
> ***Barrow type A:*** Direct fistula between the intracavernous ICA and the cavernous sinus
> ***Barrrow type B:*** Indirect fistula between dural branches of the ICA and the cavernous sinus
> ***Barrow type C:*** Indirect fistula between dural branches of the external carotid artery (eg, the middle meningeal artery, accessory meningeal artery, internal maxillary artery, and the cavernous sinus)
> ***Barrow type D:*** Indirect fistula between dural branches of both the internal and external carotid arteries and the cavernous sinus

Drainage to the contralateral cavernous sinus by the intercavernous (circular) sinus is also common. In these patients, bilateral orbital symptoms may result as the arterialized cavernous sinuses drain to bilateral superior ophthalmic veins, although this is rare. Less commonly, there is a component of drainage to cerebral cortical veins [168,169], with cerebral venous hypertension and resulting cortical venous ischemia or infarct. Hemispheric infarct secondary to complete steal of ICA flow has also been reported [170]. The timing and severity of presenting symptoms depends on a variety of factors, including size of the arterial rent and available routes of venous drainage. Symptoms may be immediately evident, or may also appear in a delayed fashion, sometimes months to years after injury [171,172].

CT and MR imaging of patients with CCFs commonly demonstrate enlargement of the superior ophthalmic vein, and may demonstrate enlargement of other draining venous channels or indura-tion in orbital fat. These findings, however, are not specific for CCF. Additional variable findings include bulging of the lateral wall of the cavernous sinus and enlargement of extraocular muscles. MR imaging may additionally demonstrate arterial-type flow voids in the cavernous sinus, superior ophthalmic vein, or other draining veins. CTA of direct CCF, if the contrast bolus is well-timed, may demonstrate asymmetric early opacification of a cavernous sinus in arterial phase [173]; in practice, however, this is often difficult to achieve reliably. CTA may also demonstrate a wall defect corresponding to the fistula point [174]. MR angiography may demonstrate flow enhancement in the cavernous sinus; this is often best seen on source images [175].

Angiographic work-up should include selective internal carotid and external carotid injections to distinguish direct fistulas from dural arteriovenous malformations. Vertebral artery injection should

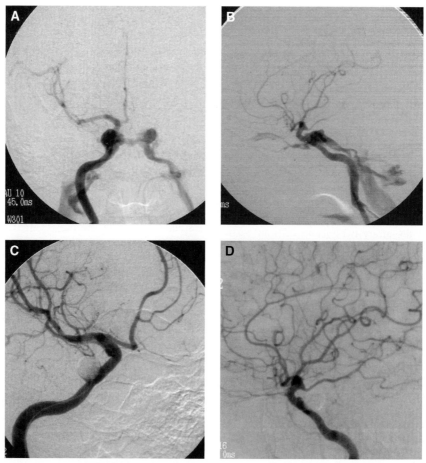

Fig. 17. CCF following motor vehicle accident. Anteroposterior (*A*) and lateral (*B*) DSA of the right ICA demonstrate a right CCF with drainage to the right superior ophthalmic vein, contralateral cavernous sinus, and bilateral inferior petrosal sinuses. (*C*) The CCF was closed with a detachable balloon placed through the fistula point, into the right cavernous sinus. (*D*) Final lateral DSA of the right ICA demonstrates complete closure of the fistula.

also be performed to evaluate collateral flow in the circle of Willis, particularly when flow to the distal ICA beyond the fistula is markedly diminished or absent. High filming rates are essential in visualizing the fistula point. Extended filming during the venous phase is also useful to assess routes of venous drainage and to evaluate whether cerebral cortical venous hypertension is present [176].

Indications for urgent treatment include (1) increased intracranial pressure or presence of cerebral cortical venous hypertension, (2) deterioration in vision, (3) increased intraocular pressure, and (4) worsening proptosis [169]. Endovascular occlusion of the fistula with preservation of the parent artery is the current preferred treatment [166,177,178]. This is most commonly accomplished by transarterial balloon embolization [93,179–181], or by transvenous or transarterial coil occlusion of the cavernous sinus [**Fig. 17**] [166,177]. Stents have also been used to close the fistulous connection [182]. Where technical factors prevent endovascular repair of the fistula point, parent vessel sacrifice may be required [183].

Summary

The imaging evaluation of neurovascular injury remains a controversial but important topic. Although conventional angiography remains the gold standard, there are clearly some important advantages to cross-sectional imaging. Immediately obvious benefits include the decreased risk of complications and less resource-intensive nature of cross-sectional imaging and, with regard to CTA, the rapidity of obtaining the study. Less evident, however, are the benefits with regard to imaging interpretation. Specifically, subtle disruptions of the vessel wall may be detected that are difficult, if not impossible, to see on angiography if they are not prominent enough to alter the contrast column. Angiographic perception of irregularity to the vessel wall not only relies on this alteration of the contour or density of the contrast column, but is often dependent on the angle from which the vessel is viewed, because summation of shadows can obscure lesions. The planar reconstructions and particularly the axial source images of cross-sectional imaging studies are not as affected by this phenomenon. Regardless, cross-sectional data can be manipulated to view the vessel at any angle, not just those views chosen during the catheter study as in conventional angiography (although three-dimensional rotational angiographic ability may obviate this problem). An additional benefit of cross-sectional methods is the ability to study the surrounding tissues; the radiologist can gauge where vessels were most likely subjected to the greatest stress, and where they are most likely to have been injured. For these reasons, the use of cross-sectional imaging studies will likely continue to grow as an important tool in the evaluation of this patient population. The modality does, however, have limitations that become evident when trying to visualize the vessels as they traverse bony foramina or course adjacent to metallic fragments; conventional digital subtraction angiography is typically not as affected by these difficulties.

A wide variety of types of injury have been presented, with equally diverse clinical scenarios and potential treatment plans. The basic concept the radiologist can use in thinking about neurovascular trauma, however, is simple and threefold: (1) these lesions reflect a spectrum of degrees of injury to the vessel wall, (2) imaging features depend on the extent of damage to the wall, and (3) treatment considerations are largely determined by whether or not the wall is sufficiently intact to contain contrast and blood.

References

[1] Cothren CC, Moore EE, Biffl WL, et al. Anticoagulation is the gold standard therapy for blunt carotid injuries to reduce stroke rate. Arch Surg 2004;139:540–5 [discussion: 545–6].

[2] Biffl WL, Moore EE, Elliott JP, et al. The devastating potential of blunt vertebral arterial injuries. Ann Surg 2000;231:672–81.

[3] Biffl WL, Moore EE, Ryu RK, et al. The unrecognized epidemic of blunt carotid arterial injuries: early diagnosis improves neurologic outcome. Ann Surg 1998;228:462–70.

[4] Fabian TC, Patton Jr JH, Croce MA, et al. Blunt carotid injury: importance of early diagnosis and anticoagulant therapy. Ann Surg 1996;223: 513–22 [discussion: 522–5].

[5] Kraus RR, Bergstein JM, DeBord JR. Diagnosis, treatment, and outcome of blunt carotid arterial injuries. Am J Surg 1999;178:190–3.

[6] Sclafani SJ, Cavaliere G, Atweh N, et al. The role of angiography in penetrating neck trauma. J Trauma 1991;31:557–62 [discussion: 562–3].

[7] Snyder III WH, Thal ER, Bridges RA, et al. The validity of normal arteriography in penetrating trauma. Arch Surg 1978;113:424–6.

[8] Willinsky RA, Taylor SM, TerBrugge K, et al. Neurologic complications of cerebral angiography: prospective analysis of 2,899 procedures and review of the literature. Radiology 2003; 227:522–8.

[9] Heiserman JE, Dean BL, Hodak JA, et al. Neurologic complications of cerebral angiography. AJNR Am J Neuroradiol 1994;15:1401–7 [discussion: 1408–11].

[10] James CA. Magnetic resonance angiography in trauma. Clin Neurosci 1997;4:137–45.

[11] Bok AP, Peter JC. Carotid and vertebral artery occlusion after blunt cervical injury: the role of

MR angiography in early diagnosis. J Trauma 1996;40:968–72.

[12] Klufas RA, Hsu L, Barnes PD, et al. Dissection of the carotid and vertebral arteries: imaging with MR angiography. AJR Am J Roentgenol 1995;164:673–7.

[13] Friedman D, Flanders A, Thomas C, et al. Vertebral artery injury after acute cervical spine trauma: rate of occurrence as detected by MR angiography and assessment of clinical consequences. AJR Am J Roentgenol 1995;164:443–7 [discussion: 448–9].

[14] Sue DE, Brant-Zawadzki MN, Chance J. Dissection of cranial arteries in the neck: correlation of MRI and arteriography. Neuroradiology 1992;34:273–8.

[15] Munera F, Cohn S, Rivas LA. Penetrating injuries of the neck: use of helical computed tomographic angiography. J Trauma 2005;58:413–8.

[16] Berne JD, Norwood SH, McAuley CE, et al. Helical computed tomographic angiography: an excellent screening test for blunt cerebrovascular injury. J Trauma 2004;57:11–7 [discussion: 17].

[17] Miller PR, Fabian TC, Croce MA, et al. Prospective screening for blunt cerebrovascular injuries: analysis of diagnostic modalities and outcomes. Ann Surg 2002;236:386–93 [discussion: 393–5].

[18] Munera F, Soto JA, Palacio DM, et al. Penetrating neck injuries: helical CT angiography for initial evaluation. Radiology 2002;224:366–72.

[19] Munera F, Soto JA, Palacio D, et al. Diagnosis of arterial injuries caused by penetrating trauma to the neck: comparison of helical CT angiography and conventional angiography. Radiology 2000;216:356–62.

[20] Ramadan F, Rutledge R, Oller D, et al. Carotid artery trauma: a review of contemporary trauma center experiences. J Vasc Surg 1995;21:46–55 [discussion: 55–6].

[21] du Toit DF, van Schalkwyk GD, Wadee SA, et al. Neurologic outcome after penetrating extracranial arterial trauma. J Vasc Surg 2003;38:257–62.

[22] Miller PR, Fabian TC, Bee TK, et al. Blunt cerebrovascular injuries: diagnosis and treatment. J Trauma 2001;51:279–85 [discussion: 285–6].

[23] Carrillo EH, Osborne DL, Spain DA, et al. Blunt carotid artery injuries: difficulties with the diagnosis prior to neurologic event. J Trauma 1999;46:1120–5.

[24] Alimi Y, Di Mauro P, Tomachot L, et al. Bilateral dissection of the internal carotid artery at the base of the skull due to blunt trauma: incidence and severity. Ann Vasc Surg 1998;12:557–65.

[25] Sclafani AP, Sclafani SJ. Angiography and transcatheter arterial embolization of vascular injuries of the face and neck. Laryngoscope 1996;106(2 Pt 1):168–73.

[26] Cogbill TH, Moore EE, Meissner M, et al. The spectrum of blunt injury to the carotid artery: a multicenter perspective. J Trauma 1994;37:473–9.

[27] Martin RF, Eldrup-Jorgensen J, Clark DE, et al. Blunt trauma to the carotid arteries. J Vasc Surg 1991;14:789–93 [discussion: 793–5].

[28] Davis JW, Holbrook TL, Hoyt DB, et al. Blunt carotid artery dissection: incidence, associated injuries, screening, and treatment. J Trauma 1990;30:1514–7.

[29] Krajewski LP, Hertzer NR. Blunt carotid artery trauma: report of two cases and review of the literature. Ann Surg 1980;191:341–6.

[30] Perry MO, Snyder WH, Thal ER. Carotid artery injuries caused by blunt trauma. Ann Surg 1980;192:74–7.

[31] Yamada S, Kindt GW, Youmans JR. Carotid artery occlusion due to nonpenetrating injury. J Trauma 1967;7:333–42.

[32] Lucas C, Moulin T, Deplanque D, et al. Stroke patterns of internal carotid artery dissection in 40 patients. Stroke 1998;29:2646–8.

[33] Diaz-Daza O, Arraiza FJ, Barkley JM, et al. Endovascular therapy of traumatic vascular lesions of the head and neck. Cardiovasc Intervent Radiol 2003;26:213–21.

[34] Biffl WL, Moore EE, Offner PJ, et al. Blunt carotid arterial injuries: implications of a new grading scale. J Trauma 1999;47:845–53.

[35] Rao PM, Ivatury RR, Sharma P, et al. Cervical vascular injuries: a trauma center experience. Surgery 1993;114:527–31.

[36] Mokri B, Sundt Jr TM, Houser OW, et al. Spontaneous dissection of the cervical internal carotid artery. Ann Neurol 1986;19:126–38.

[37] Schievink WI, Mokri B, Garrity JA, et al. Ocular motor nerve palsies in spontaneous dissections of the cervical internal carotid artery. Neurology 1993;43:1938–41.

[38] Mokri B, Schievink WI, Olsen KD, et al. Spontaneous dissection of the cervical internal carotid artery: presentation with lower cranial nerve palsies. Arch Otolaryngol Head Neck Surg 1992;118:431–5.

[39] Kerwin AJ, Bynoe RP, Murray J, et al. Liberalized screening for blunt carotid and vertebral artery injuries is justified. J Trauma 2001;51:308–14.

[40] Fabian TC, George Jr SM, Croce MA, et al. Carotid artery trauma: management based on mechanism of injury. J Trauma 1990;30:953–61 [discussion: 961–3].

[41] Zimmerman RA, Bilaniuk LT, Gennarelli T, et al. Cranial computed tomography in diagnosis and management of acute head trauma. AJR Am J Roentgenol 1978;131:27–34.

[42] Paterakis K, Karantanas AH, Komnos A, et al. Outcome of patients with diffuse axonal injury: the significance and prognostic value of MRI in the acute phase. J Trauma 2000;49:1071–5.

[43] Kelly AB, Zimmerman RD, Snow RB, et al. Head trauma: comparison of MR and CT: experience

in 100 patients. AJNR Am J Neuroradiol 1988;9: 699–708.

[44] Snow RB, Zimmerman RD, Gandy SE, et al. Comparison of magnetic resonance imaging and computed tomography in the evaluation of head injury. Neurosurgery 1986;18:45–52.

[45] Nemzek WR, Hecht ST, Donald PJ, et al. Prediction of major vascular injury in patients with gunshot wounds to the neck. AJNR Am J Neuroradiol 1996;17:161–7.

[46] York G, Barboriak D, Petrella J, et al. Association of internal carotid artery injury with carotid canal fractures in patients with head trauma. AJR Am J Roentgenol 2005;184:1672–8.

[47] Veras LM, Pedraza-Gutierrez S, Castellanos J, et al. Vertebral artery occlusion after acute cervical spine trauma. Spine 2000;25:1171–7.

[48] Willis BK, Greiner F, Orrison WW, et al. The incidence of vertebral artery injury after mid-cervical spine fracture or subluxation. Neurosurgery 1994;34:435–41 [discussion: 441–2].

[49] Parent AD, Harkey HL, Touchstone DA, et al. Lateral cervical spine dislocation and vertebral artery injury. Neurosurgery 1992;31:501–9.

[50] Schwarz N, Buchinger W, Gaudernak T, et al. Injuries to the cervical spine causing vertebral artery trauma: case reports. J Trauma 1991;31: 127–33.

[51] Louw JA, Mafoyane NA, Small B, et al. Occlusion of the vertebral artery in cervical spine dislocations. J Bone Joint Surg Br 1990;72: 679–81.

[52] Yang WG, Chen CT, de Villa GH, et al. Blunt internal carotid artery injury associated with facial fractures. Plast Reconstr Surg 2003;111: 789–96.

[53] Fabian TS, Woody JD, Ciraulo DL, et al. Post-traumatic carotid cavernous fistula: frequency analysis of signs, symptoms, and disability outcomes after angiographic embolization. J Trauma 1999;47:275–81.

[54] Goodwin JR, Johnson MH. Carotid injury secondary to blunt head trauma: case report. J Trauma 1994;37:119–22.

[55] O'Sullivan RM, Graeb DA, Nugent RA, et al. Carotid and vertebral artery trauma: clinical and angiographic features. Australas Radiol 1991; 35:47–55.

[56] Fiebach J, Jansen O, Schellinger P, et al. Comparison of CT with diffusion-weighted MRI in patients with hyperacute stroke. Neuroradiology 2001;43:628–32.

[57] Lansberg MG, Albers GW, Beaulieu C, et al. Comparison of diffusion-weighted MRI and CT in acute stroke. Neurology 2000;54:1557–61.

[58] Schaefer PW, Huisman TA, Sorensen AG, et al. Diffusion-weighted MR imaging in closed head injury: high correlation with initial Glasgow coma scale score and score on modified Rankin scale at discharge. Radiology 2004;233:58–66.

[59] Pittella JE, Gusmao SN. Diffuse vascular injury in fatal road traffic accident victims: its rela-

tionship to diffuse axonal injury. J Forensic Sci 2003;48:626–30.

[60] Shah GV, Quint DJ, Trobe JD. Magnetic resonance imaging of suspected cervicocranial arterial dissections. J Neuroophthalmol 2004; 24:315–8.

[61] LeBlang SD, Nunez Jr DB, Rivas LA, et al. Helical computed tomography in penetrating neck trauma. Emerg Radiol 1997;4:200–6.

[62] Mascalchi M, Bianchi MC, Mangiafico S, et al. MRI and MR angiography of vertebral artery dissection. Neuroradiology 1997;39:329–40.

[63] Nunez Jr DB, Torres-Leon M, Munera F. Vascular injuries of the neck and thoracic inlet: helical CT-angiographic correlation. Radiographics 2004;24:1087–98 [discussion: 1099–100].

[64] Munera F, Soto JA, Nunez D. Penetrating injuries of the neck and the increasing role of CTA. Emerg Radiol 2004;10:303–9.

[65] Ohtsuka K, Hashimoto M. The results of serial dynamic enhanced computed tomography in patients with carotid-cavernous sinus fistulas. Jpn J Ophthalmol 1999;43:559–64.

[66] Krings T, Hans F. New developments in MRA: time-resolved MRA. Neuroradiology 2004; 46(Suppl 2):s214–22.

[67] Nason RW, Assuras GN, Gray PR, et al. Penetrating neck injuries: analysis of experience from a Canadian trauma centre. Can J Surg 2001;44:122–6.

[68] Bumpous JM, Whitt PD, Ganzel TM, et al. Penetrating injuries of the visceral compartment of the neck. Am J Otolaryngol 2000;21:190–4.

[69] Demetriades D, Theodorou D, Cornwell E, et al. Evaluation of penetrating injuries of the neck: prospective study of 223 patients. World J Surg 1997;21:41–7 [discussion: 47–8].

[70] Ginzburg E, Montalvo B, LeBlang S, et al. The use of duplex ultrasonography in penetrating neck trauma. Arch Surg 1996;131:691–3.

[71] Amato JJ, Billy LJ, Gruber RP, et al. Vascular injuries: an experimental study of high and low velocity missile wounds. Arch Surg 1970;101: 167–74.

[72] Golueke P, Sclafani S, Phillips T, et al. Vertebral artery injury: diagnosis and management. J Trauma 1987;27:856–65.

[73] Sclafani SJ, Scalea TM, Wetzel W, et al. Internal carotid artery gunshot wounds. J Trauma 1996; 40:751–7.

[74] Mullins ME, Schaefer PW, Sorensen AG, et al. CT and conventional and diffusion-weighted MR imaging in acute stroke: study in 691 patients at presentation to the emergency department. Radiology 2002;224:353–60.

[75] Kloska SP, Nabavi DG, Gaus C, et al. Acute stroke assessment with CT: do we need multi-modal evaluation? Radiology 2004;233:79–86.

[76] Smith AS, Hurst GC, Duerk JL, et al. MR of ballistic materials: imaging artifacts and potential hazards. AJNR Am J Neuroradiol 1991;12: 567–72.

[77] Hollerman JJ, Fackler ML, Coldwell DM, et al. Gunshot wounds: 2. Radiology. AJR Am J Roentgenol 1990;155:691–702.

[78] Gracias VH, Reilly PM, Philpott J, et al. Computed tomography in the evaluation of penetrating neck trauma: a preliminary study. Arch Surg 2001;136:1231–5.

[79] Ofer A, Nitecki SS, Braun J, et al. CT angiography of the carotid arteries in trauma to the neck. Eur J Vasc Endovasc Surg 2001;21: 401–7.

[80] Schievink WI. The treatment of spontaneous carotid and vertebral artery dissections. Curr Opin Cardiol 2000;15:316–21.

[81] Davis JW, Holbrook TL, Hoyt DB, et al. Blunt carotid artery dissection: incidence, associated injuries, screening, and treatment. J Trauma 1990; 30:1514–7.

[82] Mittal VK, Paulson TJ, Colaiuta E, et al. Carotid artery injuries and their management. J Cardiovasc Surg (Torino) 2000;41:423–31.

[83] Beletsky V, Nadareishvili Z, Lynch J, et al. Cervical arterial dissection: time for a therapeutic trial? Stroke 2003;34:2856–60.

[84] Lyrer P, Engelter S. Antithrombotic drugs for carotid artery dissection. Cochrane Database Syst Rev 2003;3:CD000255.

[85] Redekop G, Marotta T, Weill A. Treatment of traumatic aneurysms and arteriovenous fistulas of the skull base by using endovascular stents. J Neurosurg 2001;95:412–9.

[86] Hemphill III JC, Gress DR, Halbach VV. Endovascular therapy of traumatic injuries of the intracranial cerebral arteries. Crit Care Clin 1999; 15:811–29.

[87] Bejjani GK, Monsein LH, Laird JR, et al. Treatment of symptomatic cervical carotid dissections with endovascular stents. Neurosurgery 1999;44:755–60 [discussion: 760–1].

[88] Felber S, Henkes H, Weber W, et al. Treatment of extracranial and intracranial aneurysms and arteriovenous fistulae using stent grafts. Neurosurgery 2004;55:631–8. [discussion: 638–9].

[89] Assadian A, Senekowitsch C, Rotter R, et al. Long-term results of covered stent repair of internal carotid artery dissections. J Vasc Surg 2004;40:484–7.

[90] Kubaska III SM, Greenberg RK, Clair D, et al. Internal carotid artery pseudoaneurysms: treatment with the Wallgraft endoprosthesis. J Endovasc Ther 2003;10:182–9.

[91] McNeil JD, Chiou AC, Gunlock MG, et al. Successful endovascular therapy of a penetrating zone III internal carotid injury. J Vasc Surg 2002;36:187–90.

[92] Vinchon M, Laurian C, George B, et al. Vertebral arteriovenous fistulas: a study of 49 cases and review of the literature. Cardiovasc Surg 1994; 2:359–69.

[93] Higashida RT, Halbach VV, Tsai FY, et al. Interventional neurovascular treatment of traumatic carotid and vertebral artery lesions: results in 234 cases. AJR Am J Roentgenol 1989;153: 577–82.

[94] Ben-Menachem Y, Fields WS, Cadavid G, et al. Vertebral artery trauma: transcatheter embolization. AJNR Am J Neuroradiol 1987;8:501–7.

[95] Prall JA, Brega KE, Coldwell DM, et al. Incidence of unsuspected blunt carotid artery injury. Neurosurgery 1998;42:495–8 [discussion: 498–9].

[96] Bendixen BH, Posner J, Lango R. Stroke in young adults and children. Curr Neurol Neurosci Rep 2001;1:54–66.

[97] Malm J, Kristensen B, Carlberg B, et al. Clinical features and prognosis in young adults with infratentorial infarcts. Cerebrovasc Dis 1999;9: 282–9.

[98] Kasantikul V, Ouellet JV, Smith TA. Head and neck injuries in fatal motorcycle collisions as determined by detailed autopsy. Traffic Inj Prev 2003;4:255–62.

[99] Smith WS, Johnston SC, Skalabrin EJ, et al. Spinal manipulative therapy is an independent risk factor for vertebral artery dissection. Neurology 2003;60:1424–8.

[100] Nadgir RN, Loevner LA, Ahmed T, et al. Simultaneous bilateral internal carotid and vertebral artery dissection following chiropractic manipulation: case report and review of the literature. Neuroradiology 2003;45:311–4.

[101] Rothwell DM, Bondy SJ, Williams JI. Chiropractic manipulation and stroke: a population-based case-control study. Stroke 2001;32:1054–60.

[102] Hufnagel A, Hammers A, Schonle PW, et al. Stroke following chiropractic manipulation of the cervical spine. J Neurol 1999;246:683–8.

[103] Lee KP, Carlini WG, McCormick GF, et al. Neurologic complications following chiropractic manipulation: a survey of California neurologists. Neurology 1995;45:1213–5.

[104] Pary LF, Rodnitzky RL. Traumatic internal carotid artery dissection associated with taekwondo. Neurology 2003;60:1392–3.

[105] McCrory P. Vertebral artery dissection causing stroke in sport. J Clin Neurosci 2000;7:298–300.

[106] Schievink WI, Atkinson JL, Bartleson JD, et al. Traumatic internal carotid artery dissections caused by blunt softball injuries. Am J Emerg Med 1998;16:179–82.

[107] Lannuzel A, Moulin T, Amsallem D, et al. Vertebral-artery dissection following a judo session: a case report. Neuropediatrics 1994; 25:106–8.

[108] Tramo MJ, Hainline B, Petito F, et al. Vertebral artery injury and cerebellar stroke while swimming: case report. Stroke 1985;16:1039–42.

[109] Rogers L, Sweeney PJ. Stroke: a neurologic complication of wrestling. A case of brainstem stroke in a 17-year-old athlete. Am J Sports Med 1979;7:352–4.

[110] Egnor MR, Page LK, David C. Vertebral artery aneurysm: a unique hazard of head banging by heavy metal rockers. Case report. Pediatr Neurosurg 1991–92;17:135–8.

[111] Traflet RF, Babaria AR, Bell RD, et al. Vertebral artery dissection after rapid head turning. AJNR Am J Neuroradiol 1989;10:650–1.

[112] Bush RL, Lin PH, Dodson TF, et al. Endoluminal stent placement and coil embolization for the management of carotid artery pseudoaneurysms. J Endovasc Ther 2001;8:53–61.

[113] Malek AM, Higashida RT, Phatouros CC, et al. Endovascular management of extracranial carotid artery dissection achieved using stent angioplasty. AJNR Am J Neuroradiol 2000;21: 1280–92.

[114] Kerby JD, May AK, Gomez CR, et al. Treatment of bilateral blunt carotid injury using percutaneous angioplasty and stenting: case report and review of the literature. J Trauma 2000; 49:784–7.

[115] Coldwell DM, Novak Z, Ryu RK, et al. Treatment of posttraumatic internal carotid arterial pseudoaneurysms with endovascular stents. J Trauma 2000;48:470–2.

[116] Simionato F, Righi C, Scotti G. Post-traumatic dissecting aneurysm of extracranial internal carotid artery: endovascular treatment with stenting. Neuroradiology 1999;41:543–7.

[117] Matsuura JH, Rosenthal D, Jerius H, et al. Traumatic carotid artery dissection and pseudoaneurysm treated with endovascular coils and stent. J Endovasc Surg 1997;4:339–43.

[118] Perez-Cruet MJ, Patwardhan RV, Mawad ME, et al. Treatment of dissecting pseudoaneurysm of the cervical internal carotid artery using a wall stent and detachable coils: case report. Neurosurgery 1997;40:622–5 [discussion: 625–6].

[119] Cothren CC, Moore EE, Ray Jr CE, et al. Carotid artery stents for blunt cerebrovascular injury: risks exceed benefits. Arch Surg 2005;140: 480–5 [discussion: 485–6].

[120] Yadav JS, Wholey MH, Kuntz RE, et al. Protected carotid-artery stenting versus endarterectomy in high-risk patients. N Engl J Med 2004;351:1493–501.

[121] Liu AY, Paulsen RD, Marcellus ML, et al. Long-term outcomes after carotid stent placement treatment of carotid artery dissection. Neurosurgery 1999;45:1368–73 [discussion: 1373–4].

[122] Halbach VV, Higashida RT, Hieshima GB. Treatment of vertebral arteriovenous fistulas. AJR Am J Roentgenol 1988;150:405–12.

[123] Duncan IC, Fourie PA. Percutaneous management of concomitant post-traumatic high vertebrovertebral and caroticojugular fistulas using balloons, coils, and a covered stent. J Endovasc Ther 2003;10:882–6.

[124] Hung CL, Wu YJ, Lin CS, et al. Sequential endovascular coil embolization for a traumatic cervical vertebral AV fistula. Catheter Cardiovasc Interv 2003;60:267–9.

[125] Kypson AP, Wentzensen N, Georgiade GS, et al. Traumatic vertebrojugular arteriovenous fistula: case report. J Trauma 2000;49:1141–3.

[126] Jansen O, Dorfler A, Forsting M, et al. Endovascular therapy of arteriovenous fistulae with electrolytically detachable coils. Neuroradiology 1999;41:951–7.

[127] Amirjamshidi A, Abbassioun K, Rahmat H. Traumatic aneurysms and arteriovenous fistulas of the extracranial vessels in war injuries. Surg Neurol 2000;53:136–45.

[128] Robbs JV, Carrim AA, Kadwa AM, et al. Traumatic arteriovenous fistula: experience with 202 patients. Br J Surg 1994;81:1296–9.

[129] Self ML, Mangram A, Jefferson H, et al. Percutaneous stent-graft repair of a traumatic common carotid-internal jugular fistula and pseudoaneurysm in a patient with cervical spine fractures. J Trauma 2004;57:1331–4.

[130] Ahn JY, Chung YS, Lee BH, et al. Stent-graft placement in a traumatic internal carotid-internal jugular fistula and pseudoaneurysm. J Clin Neurosci 2004;11:636–9.

[131] Ramsay DW, McAuliffe W. Traumatic pseudoaneurysm and high flow arteriovenous fistula involving internal jugular vein and common carotid artery: treatment with covered stent and embolization. Australas Radiol 2003;47:177–80.

[132] Borden NM, Dungan D, Dean BL, et al. Post-traumatic epistaxis from injury to the pterygovaginal artery. AJNR Am J Neuroradiol 1996;17: 1148–50.

[133] Rogers SN, Patel M, Beirne JC, et al. Traumatic aneurysm of the maxillary artery: the role of interventional radiology. A report of two cases. Int J Oral Maxillofac Surg 1995;24:336–9.

[134] Mehrotra ON, Brown GE, Widdowson WP, et al. Arteriography and selective embolisation in the control of life-threatening haemorrhage following facial fractures. Br J Plast Surg 1984; 37:482–5.

[135] Murakami R, Kumazaki T, Tajima H, et al. Transcatheter arterial embolization as treatment for life-threatening maxillofacial injury. Radiat Med 1996;14:197–9.

[136] Kurata A, Kitahara T, Miyasaka Y, et al. Superselective embolization for severe traumatic epistaxis caused by fracture of the skull base. AJNR Am J Neuroradiol 1993;14:343–5.

[137] Demetriades D, Chahwan S, Gomez H, et al. Initial evaluation and management of gunshot wounds to the face. J Trauma 1998;45:39–41.

[138] Borsa JJ, Fontaine AB, Eskridge JM, et al. Transcatheter arterial embolization for intractable epistaxis secondary to gunshot wounds. J Vasc Interv Radiol 1999;10:297–302.

[139] Hern JD, Coley SC, Hollis LJ, et al. Delayed massive epistaxis due to traumatic intracavernous carotid artery pseudoaneurysm. J Laryngol Otol 1998;112:396–8.

[140] Chen D, Concus AP, Halbach VV, et al. Epistaxis originating from traumatic pseudoaneurysm of the internal carotid artery: diagnosis and endovascular therapy. Laryngoscope 1998; 108:326–31.

[141] Gerbino G, Ramieri GA, Nasi A. Diagnosis and

treatment of retrobulbar haematomas following blunt orbital trauma: a description of eight cases. Int J Oral Maxillofac Surg 2005; 34:127–31.

[142] Hodes BL, Edelman D. Central retinal artery occlusion after facial trauma. Ophthalmic Surg 1979;10:21–3.

[143] Amirjamshidi A, Rahmat H, Abbassioun K. Traumatic aneurysms and arteriovenous fistulas of intracranial vessels associated with penetrating head injuries occurring during war: principles and pitfalls in diagnosis and management. A survey of 31 cases and review of the literature. J Neurosurg 1996;84:769–80.

[144] Aarabi B. Management of traumatic aneurysms caused by high-velocity missile head wounds. Neurosurg Clin N Am 1995;6:775–97.

[145] Aarabi B. Traumatic aneurysms of brain due to high velocity missile head wounds. Neurosurgery 1988;22(6 Pt 1):1056–63.

[146] Ferry Jr DJ, Kempe LG. False aneurysm secondary to penetration of the brain through orbitofacial wounds: report of two cases. J Neurosurg 1972;36:503–6.

[147] Kieck CF, de Villiers JC. Vascular lesions due to transcranial stab wounds. J Neurosurg 1984;60: 42–6.

[148] Rezai AR, Lee M, Kite C, et al. Traumatic posterior cerebral artery aneurysm secondary to an intracranial nail: case report. Surg Neurol 1994; 42:312–5.

[149] Ohta M, Matsuno H. Proximal M2 false aneurysm after head trauma: case report. Neurol Med Chir (Tokyo) 2001;41:131–4.

[150] Banfield GK, Brasher PF, Deans JA, et al. Intrapetrous carotid artery aneurysm presenting as epistaxis and otalgia. J Laryngol Otol 1995; 109:865–7.

[151] Nakstad P, Nornes H, Hauge HN. Traumatic aneurysms of the pericallosal arteries. Neuroradiology 1986;28:335–8.

[152] Levine NB, Tanaka T, Jones BV, et al. Minimally invasive management of a traumatic artery aneurysm resulting from shaken baby syndrome. Pediatr Neurosurg 2004;40:128–31.

[153] Pollanen MS, Deck JH, Blenkinsop B, et al. Fracture of temporal bone with exsanguination: pathology and mechanism. Can J Neurol Sci 1992;19:196–200.

[154] Han MH, Sung MW, Chang KH, et al. Traumatic pseudoaneurysm of the intracavernous ICA presenting with massive epistaxis: imaging diagnosis and endovascular treatment. Laryngoscope 1994;104(3 Pt 1):370–7.

[155] Alvarez JA, Bambakidis N, Takaoka Y. Delayed rupture of traumatic intracranial pseudoaneurysm in a child following gunshot wound to the head. J Craniomaxillofac Trauma 1999;5: 39–44.

[156] Horowitz MB, Kopitnik TA, Landreneau F, et al. Multidisciplinary approach to traumatic intracranial aneurysms secondary to shotgun and handgun wounds. Surg Neurol 1999;51:31–41 [discussion: 41–2].

[157] Fleischer AS, Patton JM, Tindall GT. Cerebral aneurysms of traumatic origin. Surg Neurol 1975;4:233–9.

[158] Saeed AB, Shuaib A, Al-Sulaiti G, et al. Vertebral artery dissection: warning symptoms, clinical features and prognosis in 26 patients. Can J Neurol Sci 2000;27:292–6.

[159] Levy ML, Rezai A, Masri LS, et al. The significance of subarachnoid hemorrhage after penetrating craniocerebral injury: correlations with angiography and outcome in a civilian population. Neurosurgery 1993;32:532–40.

[160] du Trevou MD, van Dellen JR. Penetrating stab wounds to the brain: the timing of angiography in patients presenting with the weapon already removed. Neurosurgery 1992;31:905–11 [discussion: 911–2].

[161] Cohen JE, Rajz G, Itshayek E, et al. Endovascular management of traumatic and iatrogenic aneurysms of the pericallosal artery: report of two cases. J Neurosurg 2005;102:555–7.

[162] Schuster JM, Santiago P, Elliott JP, et al. Acute traumatic posteroinferior cerebellar artery aneurysms: report of three cases. Neurosurgery 1999;45:1465–7 [discussion: 1467–8].

[163] Teitelbaum GP, Bernstein K, Choi S, et al. Endovascular coil occlusion of a traumatic basilar-cavernous fistula: technical report. Neurosurgery 1998;42:1394–7 [discussion: 1397–8].

[164] Barrow DL, Spector RH, Braun IF, et al. Classification and treatment of spontaneous carotid-cavernous sinus fistulas. J Neurosurg 1985;62: 248–56.

[165] Wadlington VR, Terry JB. Endovascular therapy of traumatic carotid-cavernous fistulas. Crit Care Clin 1999;15:831–54.

[166] Halbach VV, Higashida RT, Hieshima GB, et al. Transvenous embolization of direct carotid cavernous fistulas. AJNR Am J Neuroradiol 1988;9: 741–7.

[167] Lasjaunias P, Chiu M, ter Brugge K, et al. Neurological manifestations of intracranial dural arteriovenous malformations. J Neurosurg 1986; 64:724–30.

[168] Higashida RT, Halbach VV, Barnwell SL, et al. Treatment of intracranial aneurysms with preservation of the parent vessel: results of percutaneous balloon embolization in 84 patients. AJNR Am J Neuroradiol 1990;11:633–40.

[169] Halbach VV, Hieshima GB, Higashida RT, et al. Carotid cavernous fistulae: indications for urgent treatment. AJR Am J Roentgenol 1987;149: 587–93.

[170] Iida K, Uozumi T, Arita K, et al. Steal phenomenon in a traumatic carotid-cavernous fistula. J Trauma 1995;39:1015–7.

[171] Weinstein JM, Rufenacht DA, Partington CR, et al. Delayed visual loss due to trauma of the internal carotid artery. Arch Neurol 1991;48: 490–7.

[172] Cahill DW, Rao KC, Ducker TB. Delayed carotid-cavernous fistula and multiple cranial neuropathy following basal skull fracture. Surg Neurol 1981;16:17–22.

[173] Coskun O, Hamon M, Catroux G, et al. Carotid-cavernous fistulas: diagnosis with spiral CT angiography. AJNR Am J Neuroradiol 2000;21: 712–6.

[174] Anderson K, Collie DA, Capewell A. CT angiographic appearances of carotico-cavernous fistula. Clin Radiol 2001;56:514–6.

[175] Rucker JC, Biousse V, Newman NJ. Magnetic resonance angiography source images in carotid cavernous fistulas. Br J Ophthalmol 2004;88:311.

[176] Phatouros CC, Meyers PM, Dowd CF, et al. Carotid artery cavernous fistulas. Neurosurg Clin N Am 2000;11:67–84.

[177] Halbach VV, Higashida RT, Barnwell SL, et al. Transarterial platinum coil embolization of carotid-cavernous fistulas. AJNR Am J Neuroradiol 1991;12:429–33.

[178] Bavinzski G, Killer M, Gruber A, et al. Treatment of post-traumatic carotico-cavernous fistulae using electrolytically detachable coils: technical aspects and preliminary experience. Neuroradiology 1997;39:81–5.

[179] Lewis AI, Tomsick TA, Tew Jr JM. Management of 100 consecutive direct carotid-cavernous fistulas: results of treatment with detachable balloons. Neurosurgery 1995;36:239–44 [discussion: 244–5].

[180] Debrun GM, Vinuela F, Fox AJ, et al. Indications for treatment and classification of 132 carotid-cavernous fistulas. Neurosurgery 1988; 22:285–9.

[181] Goto K, Hieshima GB, Higashida RT, et al. Treatment of direct carotid cavernous sinus fistulae: various therapeutic approaches and results in 148 cases. Acta Radiol Suppl 1986; 369:576–9.

[182] Weber W, Henkes H, Berg-Dammer E, et al. Cure of a direct carotid cavernous fistula by endovascular stent deployment. Cerebrovasc Dis 2001;12:272–5.

[183] Coley SC, Pandya H, Hodgson TJ, et al. Endovascular trapping of traumatic carotid-cavernous fistulae. AJNR Am J Neuroradiol 2003; 24:1785–8.

RADIOLOGIC
CLINICS
OF NORTH AMERICA

Radiol Clin N Am 44 (2006) 41–62

Modern Emergent Stroke Imaging: Pearls, Protocols, and Pitfalls

Mark E. Mullins, MD, PhD[a,b,*,1]

Stroke remains one of the most important clinical diagnoses for which patients are referred to the radiologist for emergent imaging. Timely and accurate imaging guides admission from the emergency department or transfer to a hospital with a dedicated stroke service, triage to the intensive care unit (ICU), anticoagulation, thrombolysis, and many other forms of treatment and management. It is important to approach each patient's imaging needs logically and tailor each work-up. Moreover, it is important constantly to review the entire process for potential improvements. Time saved in getting an accurate diagnosis of stroke may indeed decrease morbidity and mortality. This article discusses the current management of stroke imaging and reviews the relevant literature.

Background

Epidemiology

Stroke is the third most common cause of death in the United States, approximating 7% and trailing only heart disease and cancer [1]. In recent years, it

a Division of Neuroradiology, Massachusetts General Hospital, Boston, MA, USA
b Department of Radiology, Harvard Medical School, Boston, MA, USA
* Division of Neuroradiology, Massachusetts General Hospital, 55 Fruit Street, GRB 285, Boston, MA 02114.
E-mail address: Mark.Mullins@emoryhealthcare.org.
1 Present address: Department of Radiology, 1364 Clifton Road NE, Atlanta, GA 30322.

0033-8389/06/$ – see front matter © 2005 Elsevier Inc. All rights reserved.
radiologic.theclinics.com

doi:10.1016/j.rcl.2005.08.002

has become evident that estimates of stroke incidence were either rising or underestimated [2]. Traditionally, the rate of stroke in the United States was thought to be 500,000 per year based on studies of patients in Rochester, Minnesota, and Framingham, Massachusetts, which were then extrapolated to larger populations. A study by Broderick and colleagues [2] in 1998 using patients in Cincinnati, Ohio, and within adjacent Kentucky indicated the incidence of stroke was more like 700,000 per year. Williams' data [3] confirmed this estimate, identifying 712,000 strokes in 1995 that increased to 783,000 in 1996. This calculation represented an overall rate for occurrence of total stroke (both initial and recurrent) to be 269 per 100,000 population per year [3]. Williams [3] hypothesized that the total increase was caused by both increasing age of the population and the population gain.

Motivations for stroke imaging

Stroke is a common disease and any radiologist involved in neuroimaging is also involved in the imaging diagnosis of stroke [4]. Not only does the disease process carry a high mortality, but also variable (but typically high) morbidity. Stroke is the leading cause of severe disability in the United States and the leading diagnosis for disposition of patients from hospitals to long-term care facilities [1]. Treatment does exist, however, for many patients [5]. There is a potential for prominent impact of radiology imaging on patient care [6].

Therapeutic window

The early diagnosis of ischemic stroke is critical to the success of therapeutic interventions, such as thrombolysis and anticoagulation. Prior studies have indicated the time-critical nature of this disease, with only a narrow therapeutic window in the first few hours following stroke ictus, and a dramatic rise in hemorrhage complications thereafter [7–20]. Diagnosis in the first 3 hours postictus provides the opportunity for intravenous or intra-arterial thrombolysis and intra-arterial clot mechanical treatment (attempts at removing the clot or breaking it into smaller pieces), which has been shown to improve outcome [12,15,16,21]. Diagnosis in the time period between 3 and 6 hours provides an opportunity for intra-arterial thrombolysis and mechanical treatment. Diagnosis in the first 12 hours provides the opportunity for administration of neuroprotective agents, which may improve outcome. Involvement of the posterior circulation, especially the basilar artery, is treated by some physicians regardless of time of onset or up until 12 to 24 hours in some practices. This is related to the potentially high mortality and mor-

bidity associated with basilar artery thrombosis. New studies are being performed to evaluate the possibility of basing treatment on imaging rather than a time window related to ictal onset, but these protocols remain strictly experimental at the time of this writing.

Snapshot of the recent history of stroke imaging

The mainstays of early stroke diagnosis are conventional noncontrast head CT (NCCT) and conventional brain MR imaging [10,19,22–28]. Some facilities routinely use MR imaging with diffusion-weighted imaging (DWI) in the detection of acute stroke [29] because it has been shown to yield improved sensitivity, negative predictive value, and accuracy compared with NCCT and conventional MR imaging [17,21]. CT angiography (CTA) of the cerebral vasculature has been promoted by some authors as a means to diagnose the vascular occlusions of acute stroke [13,14,27,30–32], especially in the hyperacute (<3 hours postictus) setting when decisions regarding intervention are paramount [11,33]. Specifically, CTA can reliably identify filling defects within the circle of Willis or its proximal tributaries (most commonly the middle cerebral artery [MCA] [34] and its branches) and parenchymal filling-perfusion defects indicative of whole-brain perfused blood volume [24]. CTA has been shown to be very useful in the diagnosis of MCA embolic stroke and predictive of infarction volume in the MCA distribution [11,30]. In contradistinction, CTA may be less useful for stroke involving the deep gray matter or brainstem [30].

Goals for stroke imaging

The theoretical goals for stroke imaging include

1. *Access to high-quality equipment:* The author's institution uses frequently updated hardware and software and places MR imaging and CT scanners in the emergency department, being both close to each other and to the patients and referring physicians so that examinations may be done in short succession.
2. *Ability to perform specialized examinations:* Multidetector row CT scanners are necessary for most modern specialized CT examinations including CTA (hereafter all CTA denotations imply an initial NCCT followed by CTA unless otherwise noted) and CT perfusion (CTP). The author's institution has a dedicated three-dimensional (3-D) laboratory with technical coverage 24 hours a day to provide maximum intensity projections, volume-rendered reconstructions, and perfusion maps. Multiplanar reformations are avail-

able automatically from many modern CT consoles. The author also reviews images on soft copy and recommends a patient archiving and communication system for subsequent image manipulation and scrolling. MR imaging including MR angiography, DWI, and perfusion-weighted imaging (PWI) is standard on most modern MR imaging devices but does necessitate at least a 1.5-T magnet strength, echo planar imaging modalities, and a power injector.

3. *Accurate and timely diagnosis:* Imaging does not benefit the patient until interpreted; the author's institution provides 24-hour coverage for consultation, protocoling, performance, and interpretation of patients' examinations. The four primary diagnostic questions are as follows:

   a. Is there an infarct (an imaging manifestation of cytotoxic edema)?

   b. Is there intracranial hemorrhage? The stroke physicians do not alter treatment based on petechial hemorrhage but that other types of hemorrhage probably alter treatment plans.

   c. Can stroke mimics, such as encephalitis or tumor, be excluded?

   d. What portion of brain is completely infarcted and what part is salvageable or manifests as brain at risk of infarction? With some variability, decreased or restricted diffusion on DWI defines the former [35] and perfusion-diffusion mismatch on PWI or CTP defines the latter.

4. *Vascular imaging:* Fisher [36] identified in 1951 that most stroke was thromboembolic and furthermore was related to atherosclerotic carotid disease of the neck. The basic philosophy yielded is to image the neck arteries when stroke is suspected (the author prefers CTA to MR angiography or ultrasound but finds that the surgeons and neurologists are most comfortable when combinations are used).

5. *Radiation control:* One should not lose sight of the need for reduction of radiation exposure to the patient [37]. Briefly, the concept of "as low as reasonably allowable" should be implemented and examinations should be clinically indicated.

6. *Cost:* Although it is difficult to prove with certainty, many clinicians believe that an accurate imaging diagnosis likely decreases overall cost to the system.

Radiology triage of the stroke patient

First, a good history (not necessarily long or detailed, just accurate and appropriate) should be obtained. A proper history improves the ability to make a correct diagnosis [38]. Does the patient's presentation sound in any way like a stroke? If so, the patient has a high likelihood of stroke (permanent) or transient ischemic attack and imaging is indicated. If stroke is possible, expedite the neuroimaging (be aggressive in terms of getting imaging quickly and appropriately). If the hospital has an available neurologist or better yet a stroke team, ask the referring physician strongly to consider calling them immediately. Time is of the essence.

Ask the referring physician, patient, or family members about symptom (ictal) onset time. In general, the patient falls into the categories listed in Box 1.

Neuroimaging directly affects the disposition of the patient from the emergency department, whether they are discharged; admitted to the regular floor or to (neuroscience) ICU; and under what service they are admitted and managed. Treatment options guided by neuroimaging include anticoagulation; thrombolysis; mannitol or steroids; blood pressure control (hypertension or hypotension); hypervolemia-hemodilution; craniotomy; and placement of an intracranial pressure-measuring device. For patients presenting in an acceptable time

---

Box 1: **Ictal symptom onset times**

1. *Undefined, unknown, or unclear onset time:* Traditionally these patients are not eligible for thrombolysis
2. *<3 hours postictus:* Intravenous thrombolysis candidate
3. *<6 hours postictus:* Intra-arterial thrombolysis candidate
4. *>6 hours postictus:* Usually the patient is not a thrombolysis candidate but this contraindication may be made more relative in the following scenarios:

   a. *Basilar artery thrombus:* lifesaving attempts are made in somewhat heroic circumstances in some of these cases, especially if the patient is young and otherwise healthy

   b. *Ictal onset time surrogates:* perfusion imaging; replacing the archetype of ictal onset time with surrogates, such as perfusion imaging, is not yet ready for front line use but is being studied and should be considered to be controversial and at best experimental under current standards of care in terms of replacing ictal onset time. It is, however, of great use in terms of understanding the patient's physiology and many believe that patient management will soon be based primarily on these modalities, following successful studies.

frame for thrombolysis, the first task of neuro-imaging (usually NCCT in most centers) is to demonstrate lack of intracranial hemorrhage and lack of large territorial infarct (usually MCA distribution) [39–42]. Contraindications for thrombolysis include but are not limited to recent head surgery, gastrointestinal bleeding, and other bleeding diatheses. For additional and more specific indications for thrombolysis with intravenous or intra-arterial medications, the reader is directed to the reviews in the reference section. All of these factors should be evaluated while the patient is getting queued up for scanning.

Protocols

Scenario classification and where to start

If the diagnosis is unknown and the scenario is non-acute or late acute, work-up typically begins with NCCT, with decisions for additional imaging based on the results. *Hyperacute* is generally meant to ex-

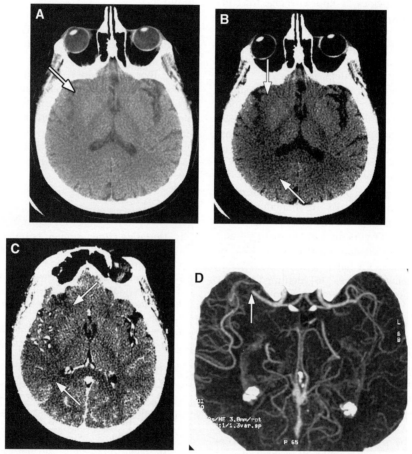

Fig. 1. A 49-year-old woman with transient ischemic attack and headache and visual field loss. (*A*) Right MCA territorial infarct is illustrated with a right insular ribbon sign on noncontrast head CT with brain windows (*arrow*) and (*B*) infarct extent better visualized using stroke windows (*arrows, border infarct extent*). (*C*) Infarct extent is also manifest on the CTA source images with stroke windows (*arrows*). (*D, E*) Right MCA clot is visualized as a filling defect on a CTA maximum intensity projection (MIP) image (*arrows*). (*F*) Axial FLAIR imaging illustrates partial infarct hyperintensity (*long arrows*) and prominent cortical vascular hyperintensity (*short arrow*), most consistent with acute infarct age. Axial DWI illustrates hyperintensity (*G*) and ADC hypointensity (*H*) within a portion of the area abnormal on CTA (*arrows*), consistent with acute infarct. (*I*) There is increased mean transit time on PWI using arterial input functions of the left internal carotid artery (ICA) (*bordered by arrows*) and (*J*) right ICA (*bordered by arrows*) (the author does not primarily use the contralateral input function because it overestimates the true abnormality but does recognize that this is controversial so both are performed). There is a similar area of decreased cerebral blood flow (*K*) that partially normalizes on the cerebral blood volume map (*L*), correlating with mean transit time maps (*short arrow, J*). This constellation of findings is most consistent with a moderate-sized infarct and a larger territory at risk for infarction, and suggestion of some, but incomplete collateralization.

press symptoms lasting fewer than 3 to 6 up until 12 hours, whereas "acute" may mean a few hours to several days, but usually means <24 hours. "Subacute" generally means several days to weeks and "chronic" means months to years (typically >3 months). The literature regarding terminology is variable, as are local usage customs. The best goal is to be descriptive, specific, and internally con-

sistent. The specific goal should be effectively to communicate the impression of the case to the referring physician.

Renal failure

If there is known or suspected renal failure in a patient not currently receiving routine dialysis, then triage of the patient to MR imaging without con-

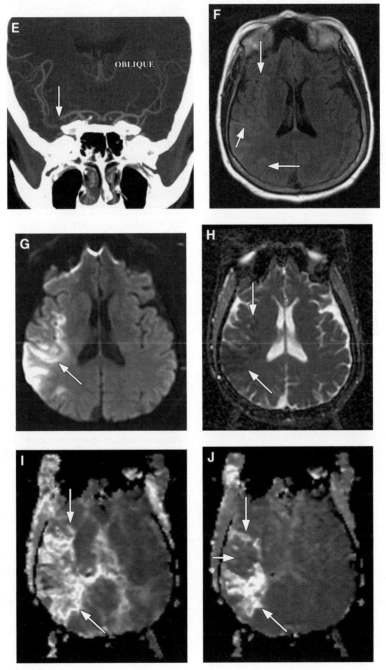

Fig. 1 (*continued*).

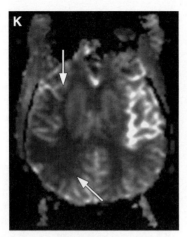
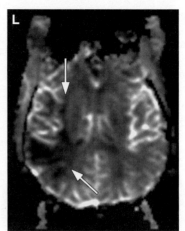

Fig. 1 (*continued*).

trast material (and without PWI) is appropriate if no other MR imaging contraindications exist. If the patient is on dialysis, then dialysis should follow in short succession any CT scan or MR image with contrast. Renal failure does not necessarily create an indication to use gadolinium-based contrast material because there are theoretical risks of heavy metal poisoning if the chelate disassociates (refer to the particular package insert for details). If the patient is to receive catheter angiography, the CTA may be obviated. The author uses creatinine values of <1.5 for normal, 1.5 to 2 for borderline (relative contraindications), and >2 for contraindication to contrast material without dialysis. In emergent circumstances, the patient's physician may approve the use of contrast material with creatinine value still pending or within the border zone region; in these cases, the risk for transient and permanent renal failure is increased. A renal medicine consult may be obtained if time allows. Use of standard medications and therapies, such as hydration and *N*-acetylcysteine, is no different than with any other patients receiving iodinated contrast material.

Access

MR imaging PWI, CTA, and contrast-enhanced MR angiography require adequate peripheral intravenous access, typically larger than 20 gauge. Larger-access cannulas are necessary for higher flow rates and access should be optimized to effect technically adequate results. Flow rates may be adjusted down for smaller access and known atrial fibrillation-arrhythmia or decreased cardiac output but the author's experience with bolus-chasing CT and MR imaging techniques has been anecdotally variable. Instead, in most instances the author simply adjusts the imaging time start point to 10 seconds

later in patients with these known diagnoses and this is sufficient to obtain interpretable images in most circumstances.

Contrast allergy

Iodinated contrast material allergy is an indication for MR imaging or MR angiography, or gadolinium-based contrast-enhanced CTA or catheter angiography. Images obtained with the latter two are typically diagnostic [43].

Hyperacute-acute stroke

For patients with hyperacute or acute stroke, the author uses CTA of the head and neck combined with CTP, followed by conventional brain MR imaging including DWI and susceptibility sequences [**Figs. 1–3**]. This version of CTA begins scanning at the skull base, extends up to the vertex, and then starts again at the arch of the aorta to complete imaging of the neck vessels. It is usually of great value to include the great artery and vertebral artery origins. Repeating arterial imaging with MR angiography after CTA is usually not indicated unless there is a problem-solving aspect to the MR angiography. T1 fat-saturated sequences for potential arterial dissection should be considered when setting up the MR imaging. If there is no territory at risk of infarction on perfusion imaging (no penumbra), it is thought that the patient is at increased risk of hemorrhage with thrombolysis; the risks of thrombolysis and mechanical intra-arterial therapy likely outweigh the benefits [**Fig. 4**]. Initial imaging should address this question.

Several different combinations of CT, MR imaging, perfusion imaging, and vascular imaging can be used to evaluate acute stroke. The author chooses initial noncontrast head CT followed immediately by CTA and CTP to provide a rapid yet thorough assessment of potential intracranial hemorrhage; stroke mimics; large evolved infarct (contraindication to thrombolysis); arterial clot and stenosis; infarct size and location; and penumbra. MR imaging adds primarily DWI, which frequently improves detail as to the presence and extent of infarct.

Many practitioners do not have quick access to MR imaging for their stroke patients and CT imaging dominates those diagnostic work-ups. Quick access to MR imaging suggests that MR imaging may also be used in lieu of CT scanning but in most situations CT scanning can be performed even before the patient is cleared and prepared for MR imaging. In some instances, more useful data can be obtained with CT methods; for example, the author finds that the increased detail in vessel imaging obtained with CT angiography is frequently more helpful than MR angiography. Because many radiologists and referring physicians believe that CT is superior to MR imaging for the assessment of intracranial hemorrhage, first-line MR imaging (in lieu of CT scanning first) remains nonstandard. In fact, MR susceptibility imaging is clearly superior to CT in identifying hemosiderin blood products that may increase the risk of intracranial hemorrhage during stroke treatment. Some data presented within the past several years have suggested that MR imaging at least as good at detecting hemorrhage, but a definitive study is indicated to convert current practice patterns. Finally, it must be re-emphasized that there is no single absolute protocol to follow and the process should be constantly re-examined for potential improvements.

Subacute stroke

For patients with subacute stroke, the author uses CTA of the head and neck without perfusion, followed by conventional brain MR imaging including DWI and susceptibility. CTP is generally not performed because most available treatments for patients in this clinical scenario do not involve perfusion data input (eg, carotid endarterectomy). There may be situations, however, in which CTP or PWI is appropriate for an individual patient.

Chronic stroke

For patients with chronic stroke the author uses conventional brain MR imaging including DWI and susceptibility combined with MR angiography of the head and neck. The author routinely performs neck MR angiography with gadolinium-based contrast material and MR angiography of the circle of Willis using 3-D time-of-flight methodology (unenhanced). Two-dimensional time-of-flight

MR angiography of the neck may complement 3-D contrast-enhanced MR angiography in some patients. Phase-contrast imaging is useful for determination of arterial flow directionality.

Neck CT angiography without noncontrast head CT

Neck CTA only (both without initial NCCT and with only a portion of the circle of Willis imaged) may be performed but the author does not recommend this option unless this is to be used for problem solving. For example, clarification of an abnormal ultrasound result is indicated.

Interpretation

Pearls

The traditional reason for performing NCCT initially is to exclude hemorrhage and obvious non-infarct disorders. Although useful in this regard, NCCT may also yield signs leading directly to a diagnosis of infarct.

In a recent study of patients, hemorrhage on NCCT was identified in approximately 5% [44]. This blood is thought to represent primarily hemorrhagic transformation of ischemic infarct. In younger patients, however, underlying vascular lesions should be considered. If a nonarterial-distribution abnormality with hemorrhage is identified, consider venous infarct. Delayed hemorrhagic conversion is most likely related to late increased arterial flow or collaterals to damaged brain (ie, reperfusion injury) or coagulopathy.

When proctoring a CTA, account for patency of the bilateral internal carotid and vertebral arteries. If there is lack of apparent contrast material filling on the initial images, the author immediately performs delayed images to see if there is delayed filling as a manifestation of hairline lumen (which usually is treated surgically) as opposed to occlusion (which likely does not undergo surgery) [45]. Anecdotally, this is at least somewhat clinically useful in every case in which it is performed.

When proctoring a CTP, consider splitting the entire contrast material bolus to cover a larger area of brain (ie, two or more scans) and be sure to include an artery in the area imaged (slab) that can be used to perform the technical aspects of the map performance (ie, arterial input function). There is controversy regarding whether to use the ipsilateral or contralateral arteries for an arterial input function and the author has chosen to use the ipsilateral artery because the contralateral artery gives an overestimate of perfusion abnormality.

If a susceptibility-weighted sequence is not available or not obtained, the author has found anecdotally that similar data may be obtained from the DWI or a subset map of apparent diffusion coefficient called *low-B* (setting the B value to nearly 0 for preparation of the map). Because the contrast on the baseline acquisition from diffusion-weighted sequences is T2 and not T2* (as in the dedicated susceptibility) sequence, it is likely that the DWI data are not optimal for detection of magnetic susceptibility artifact related to blood products; furthermore, its use has not been validated. The dedicated magnetic susceptibility (T2*) sequence is preferable [46,47].

Signs and pitfalls

Acute infarct hallmarks on routine imaging [48] include obscuration of gray-white matter interface related to cytotoxic edema; wedge-shape; vascular territorial; decreased tissue enhancement; and restricted diffusion (DWI hyperintense, apparent diffusion coefficient (ADC) hypointense, and exponential map hyperintense [49]). The intravascular enhancement sign is characteristically visible

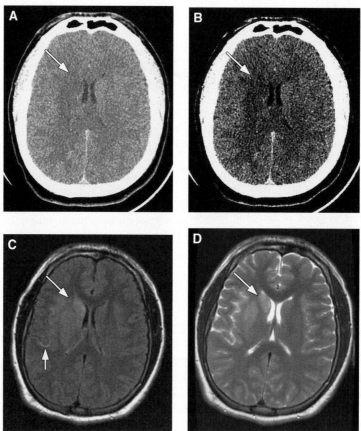

Fig. 2. A 16-year-old man with hemiparesis and neck pain. Right basal ganglia infarct (*arrows*) is illustrated with a right lentiform nucleus sign on noncontrast head CT with brain windows (*A*) and stroke windows (*B*). (*C*) Axial FLAIR imaging illustrates partial infarct hyperintensity (*long arrow*) and prominent cortical vascular hyperintensity (*short arrow*), most consistent with acute infarct age. (*D*) Axial T2-weighted imaging redemonstrates right caudate (*arrow*) and lentiform nucleus hyperintensity, most consistent with an infarct of several hours to a few days in age. An axial gradient echo susceptibility sequence image (*E*) illustrates no evidence for hemorrhagic transformation. (*F*) Postcontrast axial T1-weighted imaging illustrates intravascular enhancement (*arrow*). (*G*) Axial DWI illustrates hyperintensity (*arrow*) and (*H*) ADC hypointensity (*arrow*) within the area of abnormality on CTA, consistent with acute infarct. (*I*) Loss of flow-related enhancement is noted within a portion of the right M1segment (*between arrows*) on 3-D time-of-flight MR angiography of the circle of Willis, consistent with nonocclusive clot. (*J*) There is increased mean transit time on PWI using both in the infarcted area defined by restricted diffusion (*long arrow*), and within the posterior division territory of the right MCA (*between short arrows*), not yet infarcted based on DWI. There is an essentially matched area (*arrows*) of decreased cerebral blood flow (*K*) that only minimally normalizes on the cerebral blood volume map (*L*). This constellation of findings is most consistent with a moderate-sized completed infarct and a larger territory at risk for infarction, with incomplete collateralization.

within the first 3 days (75%), best seen on spin echo sequences and remaining one of the earliest and most sensitive signs of acute infarct [50]. This sign is relatively nonspecific, however, and resolves within 5 to 7 days, providing a narrow window of detection. The dural (meningeal) enhancement sign is best seen at the tentorium, and on coronal imaging [50]. This sign appears within the first 3 days and resolves by 7 days in most patients. Gyral enhancement of infarct is best recalled ac-

cording to Elster's rule of 3's: as early as 3 days, maximal at 3 days to 3 weeks, and gone by 3 months [50]. Use of double- or triple-dose gadolinium contrast material or use of single-dose gadolinium contrast material with magnetic transfer techniques effects earlier appearance (1 day) and a longer-lasting sign (up to 6 months) [50], although such an approach is rarely necessary.

On MR imaging, hyperintensity on T2-weighted and fluid-attenuated inversion-recovery (FLAIR)

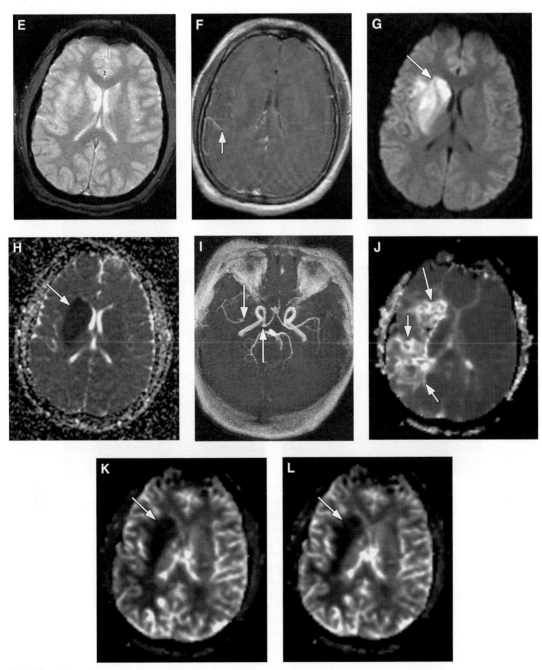

Fig. 2 (continued).

images takes several hours to a few days to develop. This observation can be useful to age an infarct. Phase and evolution hallmarks include the following milestones (caution is advised because these guidelines vary):

1. *Hyperacute infarct (<6–12 hours):* NCCT is likely normal and DWI is abnormal in approximately < 30–120 minutes and abnormality persists up to 2 weeks [35,50].
2. *Acute infarct (12–48 hours):* Meningeal enhancement, edema, and mass effect. Fogging and pseudonormalization may occur on NCCT and ADC-DWI [50].
3. *Subacute infarct (2 days–2 weeks):* Parenchymal enhancement commences at 4 days; edema resolves (maximal at 3 days); and mass effect decreases at 7 to 10 days [50]. Luxury perfusion is most evident and is likely best evidenced by increased cerebral blood volume (CBV) on PWI. In the author's experience, CBV is the most accurate initial parameter to predict outcome and final infarct volume but is not routinely obtained or necessary in the subacute setting.

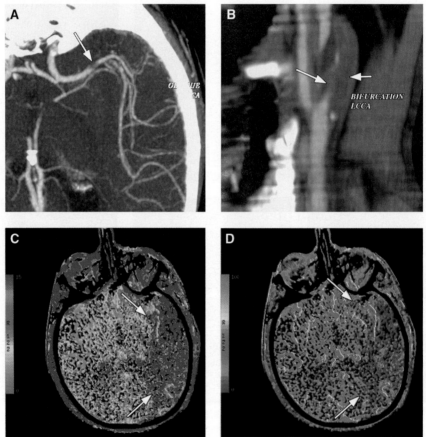

Fig. 3. A 67-year-old man with weakness. (*A*) A small, distal left MCA nonocclusive clot (*arrow*) is demonstrated on MIP reconstruction from CTA source images. (*B*) In the neck, the CTA MIP image illustrates a hairline residual lumen (*long arrow*) with atherosclerotic plaque (*short arrow*) within the proximal left cervical ICA. CTP illustrates a large area of prolonged mean transit time within the left MCA distribution (*C, arrows*), essentially matched decreased cerebral blood flow (*D, arrows*), and nearly normalized cerebral blood volume (*E*); these CTP data are most consistent with territory at risk for infarction, and good collateralization. Immediately subsequent MR imaging without thrombolysis (the patient did not meet inclusion criteria in that the ictal onset time was unclear) illustrates acute left MCA infarct on axial FLAIR (*F*) parenchymal (*between long arrows*) and cortical vessel hyperintensity (*short arrow*), no abnormal enhancement on T1-weighted imaging (not shown), no evidence for hemorrhagic transformation on susceptibility-weighted image (*G*), ill-defined and variably increased signal on DWI (*H*) and decreased on ADC maps (*I*). PWI illustrates (*J*) increased MTT (*arrow*) and (*K*) relatively matched cerebral blood flow (*arrows*) and (*L*) cerebral blood volume maps (*arrows*); this appearance is most consistent with completed infarct, which was proved on follow-up imaging (not shown). The implications of the perfusion data changed between the scans most consistent with propagation of clot. Perhaps in the future, decisions regarding thrombolysis inclusion criteria will depend more on surrogate markers, such as imaging results.

4. *Chronic infarct (>2 weeks):* Encephalomalacia (appears at 6–8 weeks) and cortical laminar necrosis [50].

Infarct signs on NCCT [51] include the following: insular ribbon sign; obscuration of the lentiform nucleus; hyperdense artery; and the MCA dot (en face) and dash sign (in profile) [52]. The author's data [52] suggest that not all dense arteries correspond to clot on CTA. Despite potential biases of CTA, it is nonetheless used for acute decision-making and the correlation to actual clot is thought to be excellent [14].

Any portion of the stroke imaging process is subject to potential pitfalls, and a few are described here. During acquisition of CTA source images it is

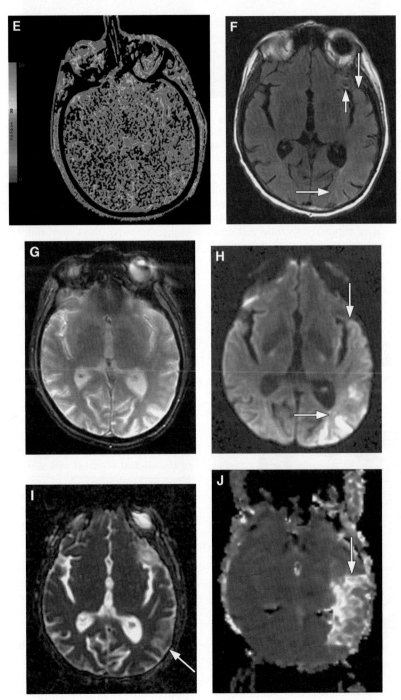

Fig. 3 (continued).

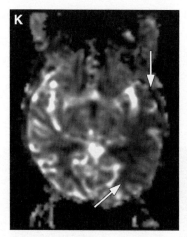
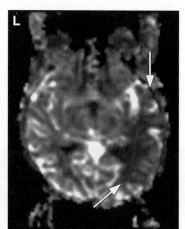

Fig. 3 (continued).

preferable to review the images quickly while the patient is still on the scanner for at least a few reasons: (1) assessment likely governs what treatment the patient receives (especially anticoagulants and thrombolytics) and any time saved may impact the results; (2) the contrast material could have extravasated and it is important to note this and treat the patient appropriately; and (3) if the typical important four vessels (bilateral internal carotid and vertebral arteries) within the neck are not opacified on all images, then delayed images may be obtained to assess whether the finding represents complete occlusion (typically not treated surgically or endovascularly) or is a critical stenosis or hairline residual lumen (treated surgically in most cases). If this is not recognized initially, additional imaging, such as sonography, catheter angiography, or MR angiography, needs to be contemplated. Another pitfall pertains to the identifi-

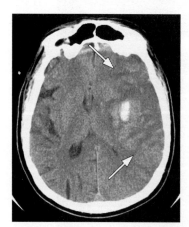

Fig. 4. A 60-year-old woman with hemiparesis. Intracranial hemorrhage is illustrated (hyperdensity) on noncontrast head CT following intra-arterial tissue plasminogen activator administered for left MCA territorial infarct (*arrows border infarct*).

cation of artifacts on CT scans and MR imaging, particularly DWI.

DWI used routinely (at 1.5-T field strength) may not identify all infarcts (false-negatives), most commonly in the posterior fossa, brainstem, and along areas near the sinuses and surface of the brain. Moreover, DWI may indicate abnormalities that eventually resolve (false-positive for infarct). These instances are sometimes related to ischemia with or without treatment but may also be seen with seizure activity and demyelination. Brain tumors may show restricted diffusion and have occasionally been mistaken for infarcts, at least initially. It is important to use all facets of the MR image characteristics to determine whether the lesion fits typical criteria across all sequences (eg, subacute infarct with T2 hyperintensity, DWI hyperintensity, ADC isointensity, possible gyral enhancement, and no mass effect). If the lesion does not demonstrate an expected appearance across all sequences, a short-term follow-up examination may be indicated to confirm expected evolution. Correlation to the clinical scenario may also benefit the diagnosis because stroke is an acute event, whereas tumor is typically insidious in onset.

A search for motion artifact on perfusion imaging should be evaluated in every case performed because the resultant perfusion maps may be erroneous and misleading, or simply uninterpretable. Evaluation of the source images using cine mode on a softcopy review system is usually helpful for evaluating the initial data before map formation and to evaluate for motion.

Infarct evaluation on angiography (CT angiography and catheter angiography)

CTA is an excellent first-line examination for evaluation of the head and neck arteries [Figs. 5 and 6]

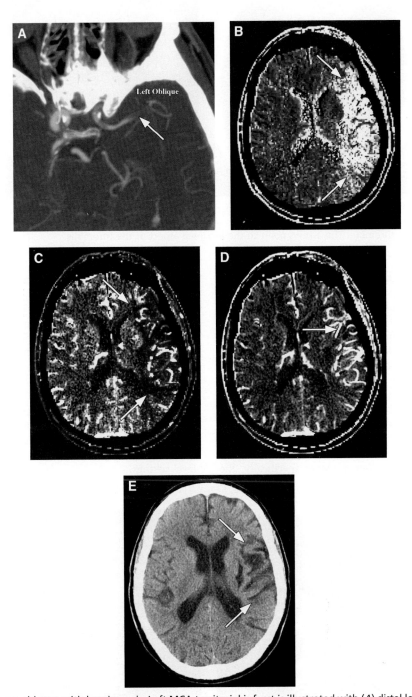

Fig. 5. A 78-year-old man with hemiparesis. Left MCA territorial infarct is illustrated with (*A*) distal left MCA filling defect consistent with thrombus (*arrow*), (*B*) increased mean transit time on CTP (*bordered by arrows*), and (*C*) a smaller area of decreased cerebral blood flow that (*D*) partially normalizes on the cerebral blood volume map. This constellation of findings is most consistent with a small infarct and a larger territory at risk for infarction, and suggestion of good collateralization. (*E*) Follow-up noncontrast head CT confirms this assessment because the final infarct volume (*between arrows*) approximates the area of infarct only on CTP, following appropriate stroke treatment (including thrombolysis).

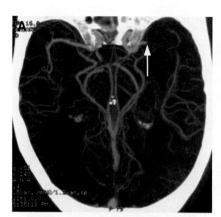
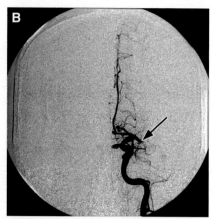

Fig. 6. A 61-year-old woman with hemiparesis. Nonocclusive left MCA thrombus on 3-D imaging performed from CTA source data (*A*) and was confirmed at catheter angiography (*B*), illustrating the typical accuracy of CTA for identification of thrombus. The arrows point to the proximal aspect of the thrombus.

[14,53]. In comparison with catheter angiography, what it gives up in resolution and dynamic properties it makes up for with rapid acquisition of a 3-D dataset and the potential for assessment of whole-brain perfusion [54] and better parenchymal evaluation [14]. Moreover, CTA illustrates not only arterial stenosis or occlusion, but also the vessel wall. This factor is most important for evaluation of intramural dissection [**Fig. 7**] and thrombosed aneurysms, which may both complicate evaluation of stroke patients.

CTA can be treated as a noninvasive angiogram, evaluating the vessels just as would be done with a conventional angiogram. More specifically, the

signs that are evaluated for both examinations include vessel occlusion or cutoff related to thromboemboli; aneurysms; arterial dissection; meniscus or flattened shape to clot (recent) versus reverse meniscus (older); tram track (nonocclusive or recanalized clot); delayed (antegrade) flow (manifest as decreased whole-brain perfusion on CTA); and (retrograde) collateral flow [55].

Use of stroke window and level settings has been shown to improve infarct detection on NCCT [**Fig. 8**] [56]. The author routinely uses these window and level settings also to evaluate CTA source images, as a supplement to routine window and level settings.

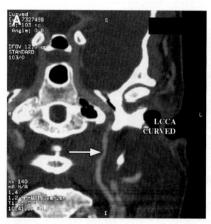
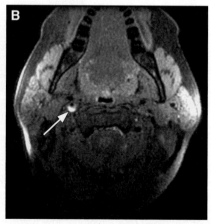

Fig. 7. A 37-year-old woman with neck pain and nonfocal clinical findings. Bilateral internal carotid artery dissections are illustrated on curved reformatted image from CTA source data (*A*) illustrating a left cervical ICA dissection (*arrow*) with smoothly tapering wall, and T1 hyperintensity within the wall of the right ICA on axial T1 noncontrast fat-saturated imaging (*B*). The left ICA abnormality is isointense on T1-weighted imaging. Findings are consistent with acute or subacute right ICA dissection (*arrow*; methemoglobin). Intensity on T1-weighted images depends on age of blood products, so the left ICA findings (isointense) could suggest either very early or chronic dissection.

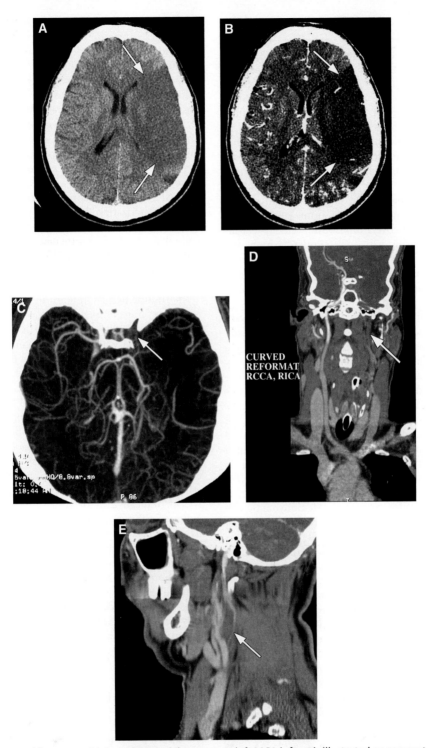

Fig. 8. A 72-year-old woman with hemiparesis. (*A*) Late acute left MCA infarct is illustrated on noncontrast head CT with brain windows (*arrows border infarct*); (*B*) noncontrast head CT with stroke windows (*arrows border infarct*); and (*C*) 3-D imaging performed from CTA source data showing a T-lesion of clot within the left ICA, M1, and A1 segments (*arrow*). The left ACA territory appears spared, suggesting that the primary arterial supply of the left ACA is not by the left A1 segment. (*D* and *E*) CTA 3-D reformatted images of the neck illustrate a severe proximal left cervical ICA stenosis (*arrow*) that includes the origin and is relatively smooth, potentially suggesting arterial dissection but more likely atherosclerotic in a patient of this age.

Factors to evaluate on CT angiography of the head and neck for stroke

Internal carotid artery stenosis [see Fig. 8] traditionally has been described by percent stenosis because of conventions used in the NASCET trials. The author, however, uses residual lumenal diameter because it more appropriately describes the physiology regardless of anatomic variations in background artery size [45]. The author describes stenoses with measurements of the smallest residual lumen and a subjective grade (mild, moderate, severe, critical). In the author's facility, 1.75-mm residual lumen corresponds to a 70% stenosis, but this may vary from laboratory to laboratory. Moreover, ultrasound velocity cutoffs for 70% stenosis vary in a similar fashion and each group must set its own standards. Previous work by the NASCET trial suggests a benefit of carotid endartarectomy for patients with symptomatic internal carotid artery stenosis >70% [57].

Identification of ulcerated plaque is also relevant because of an increased risk of thromboembolism. This diagnosis may be made to some extent on catheter angiography, but the author also routinely makes this assessment on CTA. Reporting of location of calcifications or plaque without stenosis related to atherosclerosis may benefit the patient's primary caregiver using medical management. In the future, it is likely that identification of so-called *vulnerable plaque* that is at increased risk of being a source of thromboembolic disease may be performed with such techniques as sonography, CTA, or MR angiography. This assessment, however, is not used routinely at present. Hemodynamic significance on CTA, may be inferred by observing poststenotic dilatation, and this observation is worth at least suggesting when communicating findings and their implications; however, it must be noted that this type of implication has not been definitely correlated in the literature and is strictly anecdotal. In the author's hospital, sonography results with velocity measurements are generally used in conjunction with CTA results to guide surgical planning. Furthermore, the vascular surgeons ask for performance and agreement between results of two of the following three examinations before consideration for endartarectomy: (1) sonography, (2) CTA, and (3) MR angiography.

Perfusion imaging

The primary goal of CTP and PWI is to determine potential brain (territory) at risk of infarction, which is thought to represent an ischemic penumbra that is salvageable if treated appropriately [58–63]. Several different types of maps may be computed from the raw data and a detailed dis-

cussion of the techniques and variations in these techniques is beyond the scope of this article, but the reader is encouraged to pursue additional clarification in the literature [64].

Standardized and semiautomated software is commercially available to assist in the task of forming perfusion maps. There are, however, a couple of technical points that should be made. First, motion artifact may not only cause the maps to appear uninterpretable but may also cause erroneous interpretation if this artifact is not identified. Second, there exists a controversy as to which side should be used as the arterial input function for the perfusion characterization. The author primarily uses the ipsilateral side because the data suggested that the contralateral side overestimated the potential territory at risk for infarction. Third, results may vary prominently if the user input functions are changed even slightly [64].

The routine perfusion maps that the author uses are mean transit time(similar to time to peak), cerebral blood flow, and CBV. The author's interpretation starts with the mean transit time map, because it yields typically the largest potentially abnormal area. On this map, increased signal is bad, indicative of delayed blood supply to this brain parenchyma. On the cerebral blood flow map, decreased signal is bad and is usually contained within the mean transit time abnormal region, representing delayed or decreased blood flow to the brain parenchyma through the normal antegrade arterial pathways. The CBV maps are likely the best estimate of collateral flow. Here, decreased signal is bad, indicative of delayed or decreased blood volume or flux into the brain parenchyma. CBV is likely the best predictor of final infarct volume but most patients end up with a final infarct volume somewhere between the size of the cerebral blood flow abnormality and the CBV abnormality (which is usually smaller than and contained within the cerebral blood flow abnormality). Increased signal may be obtained with luxury perfusion and reperfusion. In practice, relative or semiquantitative parametric maps are created for MR PWI instead of absolute quantitation. The processing for absolute quantitation is not trivial, and off-the-shelf software for this purpose is not widely available for MR PWI. There are, however, several vendor-supplied packages for quantitative CTP.

CTP and PWI are currently comparable, so use should be based on local access and practice customs. If the abnormal regions on CBV and cerebral blood flow are matched, this scenario likely represents completed infarct without good collaterals. If the abnormal regions on cerebral blood flow are greater than CBV, this is suggestive of some normalization and indicative of likely good collaterals; this situation is unlikely to extend to complete infarct if treated appropriately and aggressively. This patient is likely the best candidate for therapy. If the abnormal regions on mean transit time are greater than cerebral blood flow or CBV, no one has shown for certain what the area abnormal on mean transit time mean transit time only represents, but some clinicians treat this as potential territory at risk for infarction. If there is a perfusion deficit of any kind and the patient has hypotension or hypoxia, these regions may become ischemic or infarcted. If an area of restricted diffusion on DWI is matched to the perfusion abnormality, this scenario likely represents a completed infarct. A caveat must be made, however, that DWI can reverse rarely and although some think of restricted diffusion as infarcted tissue, there is controversy as to what portion of these cases manifest ischemia. Conversely, where there is a DWI-PWI mismatch, this likely represents brain tissue at risk [51] for infarction.

Assessment of the findings: synthesis and putative etiologies

Prognosis, risk of recurrence, and management options are influenced by stroke subtype. Most ischemic infarcts are thromboembolic, but the etiology is not always clear on clinical examination. Augmenting clinical evaluation with neuroimaging methods, such as those described previously, can be helpful in categorizing etiology into one of five subsets: (1) cardioembolic; (2) large-vessel stenotic-occlusive; (3) small-vessel occlusive; (4) other, but determined cause (eg, arterial dissection, vasculitis, and so forth); and (5) cryptogenic [65,66]. Visualizing the vessels (and often the heart and aortic arch) is a critical part of this process. In addition,

the pattern of ischemia-infarction in the brain can provide clues to etiology.

For example, infarcts of different ages but in the same region with a stuttering clinical course is suggestive of large-vessel stenosis, whereas infarcts of different ages in different arterial territories is more suggestive of a central embolic etiology, perhaps cardiac. Infarcts of the same age involving different arterial territories suggest a central embolic source [Fig. 9], again usually related to the heart, aortic arch, or perhaps a right-to-left shunt. Multiple small, primarily cortical infarcts of similar age or different ages could suggest a systemic process, such as vasculitis, but could also have a proximal embolic etiology like endocarditis. Borderzone or watershed infarct patterns might suggest a proximal embolus or large-vessel stenosis complicated by hypotension, or a combination of these. More diffuse and symmetric injury patterns are seen with global hypoxia or anoxia, such as in the setting of prolonged cardiac arrest. In practice, the exact etiology is not always clear, and combinations of patterns may be present.

The combination of anterior and middle cerebral infarcts (ACA and MCA, respectively) infarcts is suggestive of an internal carotid artery clot (also known as a *T-lesion* [Fig. 10]), a lesion with a poor prognosis. In a patient with an embolus to the MCA, infarction of the lentiform nucleus suggests a proximal M1 clot (also known as a *stem clot*) and its absence suggests clot distal to the lateral lenticulostriate arteries. Circle of Willis variants can modify the pattern of ischemia. For example, presence of large posterior communicating arteries may explain involvement of anterior and posterior circulation territories from a single embolic event through the internal carotid artery, and a

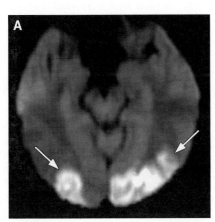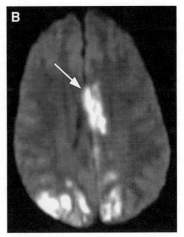

Fig. 9. A 54-year-old man with visual complaints and atrial fibrillation. Embolic acute infarcts are manifested on DWI by hyperintensities within the occipital (*arrows*), PCA territories bilaterally (*A*) and parietal, PCA territories bilaterally and the left frontal (*arrow*) ACA territory (*B*).

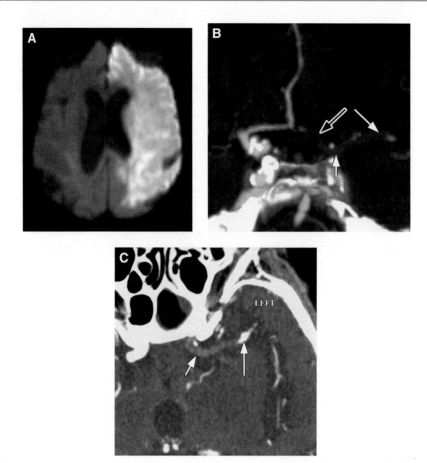

Fig. 10. A 59-year-old woman with hemiparesis. Similar situation to **Fig. 8** but in this case the left ACA territory has infarcted (*A*), whereas the right ACA territory is spared, indicating more balanced circle of Willis configuration. T-lesion is again illustrated on the left on 3-D imaging performed from CTA source data. (*B*) ICA clot (*short arrow*); M1 clot (*long arrow*); A1 clot (*open arrow*). (*C*) Left M1 clot (*short arrow*); left MCA calcified embolus versus atherosclerosis (*long arrow*).

small or absent contralateral A1 segment can lead to bilateral ACA territory infarcts from a unilateral proximal embolus like an internal carotid artery occlusion or T lesion. In general, lacunar infarcts are unlikely to be embolic, but this remains theoretically possible. In patients with lacunar infarcts, check for signs of hypertension and atherosclerotic disease on imaging, including tortuous arteries in the neck and signs of leukoaraiosis (also known as *nonspecific white matter change*).

Stroke follow-up imaging

The following are the primary aspects to be evaluated on follow-up imaging of patients with stroke (in most cases, this is accomplished with NCCT [**Fig. 11**]):

1. Has there been extension of previous infarct?
2. Is there any new location of infarct?
3. Has there been hemorrhagic transformation?
4. If there was previous hemorrhage, has it increased?
5. Has there been bleeding away from infarct?
6. Is there hydrocephalus?
7. Is there cerebral edema?
8. Is there brain herniation?

What imaging examination is really the best?

Detection of blood products

NCCT has an overall sensitivity of approximately 91% to 92% [50]. Decrease in accuracy with time is likely caused by evolution of blood density. FLAIR may be positive as early as 23 minutes, and yields sensitivity of 92% to 100% and specificity of 100% in small groups [50]. The T1-weighted MR imaging sequence is useful for identification of methemoglobin. Susceptibility (gradient recalled echo) sequences are most useful for identification of hemosiderin but are also useful for acute blood products.

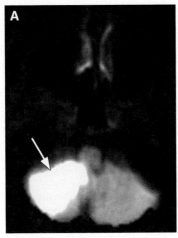
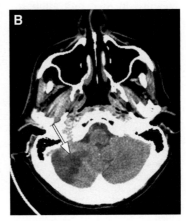

Fig. 11. A 47-year-old man with ataxia. Right PICA territory infarct (*arrow*) is illustrated on DWI (*A*) and on follow-up noncontrast head CT (*B*).

Detection of infarct

It is traditionally taught that MR imaging with DWI is superior [67–72] to NCCT and conventional MR imaging without DWI for the detection of infarct. NCCT becomes more accurate approximately 12 hours following presentation to the emergency department [72]. Data also suggest that CTA and perfusion imaging provide improvement over NCCT, with CTA placing somewhere between NCCT and MR imaging with DWI in terms of statistical values [73]. The author's results are similar to those in the literature [74–77].

Access and time of examinations

Availability of MR imaging scanners has been indicated as a limitation to the widespread use of conventional MR imaging and DWI for the diagnosis of acute stroke. CT scanners have a better penetration in the community, and may be accessed more easily and faster. Moreover, the time needed to perform NCCT followed by CTA (approximately 15 minutes) is comparable with an acute stroke protocol MR image at the author's facility. The inclusion of an MR imaging angiogram, however, nearly doubles the time of the examination for MR imaging. The inclusion of NCCT with CTA remains necessary to exclude intracranial hemorrhage, which might otherwise be overlooked because of contrast enhancement.

Summary

Stroke remains a challenge for all physicians and an important public health issue. Accurate and timely neuroimaging may affect every facet of patient care where stroke is suspected. Access to advanced CT and MR imaging techniques likely improves the ability to detect infarct and brain at risk for infarction but classical NCCT is also of use, especially where other modalities are unavailable. Because of the greater penetration of CT scanners, speed of examination, and the absence of MR imaging safety considerations with CT, CTA and CTP have become first-line evaluations of the patient with symptoms of stroke. MR imaging, and especially DWI, have become excellent diagnostic tools and may ultimately serve as first-line examinations across the United States and internationally.

References

[1] Vo KD, Lin W, Lee JM. Evidence-based neuroimaging in acute ischemic stroke. Neuroimaging Clin N Am 2003;13:167–83.

[2] Broderick J, Brott T, Kothari R, et al. The Greater Cincinnati/Northern Kentucky Stroke Study: preliminary first-ever and total incidence rates of stroke among blacks. Stroke 1998;29:415–21.

[3] Williams GR. Incidence and characteristics of total stroke in the United States. BMC Neurol 2001; 1:2.

[4] Grunwald I, Reith W. Non-traumatic neurological emergencies: imaging of cerebral ischemia. Eur Radiol 2002;12:1632–47.

[5] Albers GW, Amarenco P, Easton JD, et al. Antithrombotic and thrombolytic therapy for ischemic stroke: the Seventh ACCP Conference on Antithrombotic and Thrombolytic Therapy. Chest 2004;126:483S–512S.

[6] Rother J. CT and MRI in the diagnosis of acute stroke and their role in thrombolysis. Thromb Res 2001;103(Suppl 1):S125–33.

[7] Burnette WC, Nesbit GM, Barnwell SL. Intraarterial thrombolysis for acute stroke. Neuroimaging Clin N Am 1999;9:491–508.

[8] Jager HR. Diagnosis of stroke with advanced CT and MR imaging. Br Med Bull 2000;56: 318–33.

[9] Tegos TJ, Kalodiki E, Sabetai MM, et al. Stroke: pathogenesis, investigations, and prognosis—Part II of III. Angiology 2000;51:885–94.

[10] Kidwell CS, Villablanca JP, Saver JL. Advances in neuroimaging of acute stroke. Curr Atheroscler Rep 2000;2:126–35.

[11] Lev MH, Nichols SJ. Computed tomographic angiography and computed tomographic perfusion imaging of hyperacute stroke. Top Magn Reson Imaging 2000;11:273–87.

[12] Burnette WC, Nesbit GM. Intra-arterial thrombolysis for acute ischemic stroke. Eur Radiol 2001;11:626–34.

[13] Lev MH, Segal AZ, Farkas J, et al. Utility of perfusion-weighted CT imaging in acute middle cerebral artery stroke treated with intra-arterial thrombolysis: prediction of final infarct volume and clinical outcome. Stroke 2001;32:2021–8.

[14] Lev MH, Farkas J, Rodriguez VR, et al. CT angiography in the rapid triage of patients with hyperacute stroke to intraarterial thrombolysis: accuracy in the detection of large vessel thrombus. J Comput Assist Tomogr 2001;25:520–8.

[15] Warach S. New imaging strategies for patient selection for thrombolytic and neuroprotective therapies. Neurology 2001;57:S48–52.

[16] Laloux P. Intravenous rtPA thrombolysis in acute ischemic stroke. Acta Neurol Belg 2001; 101:88–95.

[17] Sunshine JL, Bambakidis N, Tarr RW, et al. Benefits of perfusion MR imaging relative to diffusion MR imaging in the diagnosis and treatment of hyperacute stroke. AJNR Am J Neuroradiol 2001;22:915–21.

[18] McCullough LD, Beauchamp NB, Wityk R. Recent advances in the diagnosis and treatment of stroke. Surv Ophthalmol 2001;45:317–30.

[19] Heiss WD, Forsting M, Diener HC. Imaging in cerebrovascular disease. Curr Opin Neurol 2001; 14:67–75.

[20] Keris V, Rudnicka S, Vorona V, et al. Combined intraarterial/intravenous thrombolysis for acute ischemic stroke. AJNR Am J Neuroradiol 2001; 22:352–8.

[21] Schaefer PW, Grant PE, Gonzalez RG. Diffusion-weighted MR imaging of the brain. Radiology 2000;217:331–45.

[22] Schellinger PD, Jansen O, Fiebach JB, et al. Feasibility and practicality of MR imaging of stroke in the management of hyperacute cerebral ischemia. AJNR Am J Neuroradiol 2000;21: 1184–9.

[23] Rosenwasser RH, Armonda RA. Diagnostic imaging for stroke. Clin Neurosurg 2000;46:237–60.

[24] Nakano S, Iseda T, Kawano H, et al. Correlation of early CT signs in the deep middle cerebral artery territories with angiographically confirmed site of arterial occlusion. AJNR Am J Neuroradiol 2001;22:654–9.

[25] Moonis M, Fisher M. Imaging of acute stroke. Cerebrovasc Dis 2001;11:143–50.

[26] Lee BI, Nam HS, Heo JH, et al. Yonsei Stroke Registry: analysis of 1,000 patients with acute cerebral infarctions. Cerebrovasc Dis 2001;12: 145–51.

[27] Kilpatrick MM, Yonas H, Goldstein S, et al. CT-based assessment of acute stroke: CT, CT angiography, and xenon-enhanced CT cerebral blood flow. Stroke 2001;32:2543–9.

[28] Gleason S, Furie KL, Lev MH, et al. Potential influence of acute CT on inpatient costs in patients with ischemic stroke. Acad Radiol 2001; 8:955–64.

[29] Sorensen AG, Buonanno FS, Gonzalez RG, et al. Hyperacute stroke: evaluation with combined multisection diffusion-weighted and hemodynamically weighted echo-planar MR imaging. Radiology 1996;199:391–401.

[30] Shen WC, Lee CC. Computerized tomographic angiography in the evaluation of cerebral infarction. Chung Hua I Hsueh Tsa Chih (Taipei) 1999;62:255–60.

[31] Graf J, Skutta B, Kuhn FP, et al. Computed tomographic angiography findings in 103 patients following vascular events in the posterior circulation: potential and clinical relevance. J Neurol 2000;247:760–6.

[32] Lee KH, Cho SJ, Byun HS, et al. Triphasic perfusion computed tomography in acute middle cerebral artery stroke: a correlation with angiographic findings. Arch Neurol 2000;57:990–9.

[33] Hunter GJ, Hamberg LM, Ponzo JA, et al. Assessment of cerebral perfusion and arterial anatomy in hyperacute stroke with three-dimensional functional CT: early clinical results [see comments]. AJNR Am J Neuroradiol 1998;19:29–37.

[34] Lieberman G, Abramson R, Volkan K, et al. Tutor versus computer: a prospective comparison of interactive tutorial and computer-assisted instruction in radiology education. Acad Radiol 2002;9:40–9.

[35] Burdette JH, Ricci PE, Petitti N, et al. Cerebral infarction: time course of signal intensity changes on diffusion-weighted MR images. AJR Am J Roentgenol 1998;171:791–5.

[36] Fisher CM. A career in cerebrovascular disease: a personal account. Stroke 2001;32:2719–24.

[37] Mullins ME, Lev MH, Bove P, et al. Comparison of image quality between conventional and low-dose nonenhanced head CT. AJNR Am J Neuroradiol 2004;25:533–8.

[38] Mullins ME, Lev MH, Schellingerhout D, et al. Influence of availability of clinical history on detection of early stroke using unenhanced CT and diffusion-weighted MR imaging. AJR Am J Roentgenol 2002;179:223–8.

[39] Tissue plasminogen activator for acute ischemic stroke. The National Institute of Neurological Disorders and Stroke rt-PA Stroke Study Group. N Engl J Med 1995;333:1581–7.

[40] Beauchamp Jr NJ, Barker PB, Wang PY, et al.

Imaging of acute cerebral ischemia. Radiology 1999;212:307–24.

[41] Furlan A, Higashida R, Wechsler L, et al. Intra-arterial prourokinase for acute ischemic stroke. The PROACT II study: a randomized controlled trial. Prolyse in Acute Cerebral Thromboembolism. JAMA 1999;282:2003–11.

[42] Hacke W, Kaste M, Fieschi C, et al. Intravenous thrombolysis with recombinant tissue plasminogen activator for acute hemispheric stroke. The European Cooperative Acute Stroke Study (ECASS). JAMA 1995;274:1017–25.

[43] Henson JW, Nogueira RG, Covarrubias DJ, et al. Gadolinium-enhanced CT angiography of the circle of Willis and neck. AJNR Am J Neuroradiol 2004;25:969–72.

[44] Mullins ME, Schaefer PW, Lev ML, et al. Intracranial hemorrhage complicating acute stroke in a large emergency department series: How common is it and is screening head CT necessary? In: Proceedings of the American Society of Neuroradiology (ASNR) Annual Meeting. Oak Brook (IL): ASNR; 2001. p. 321–2.

[45] Lev MH, Romero JM, Goodman DN, et al. Total occlusion versus hairline residual lumen of the internal carotid arteries: accuracy of single section helical CT angiography. AJNR Am J Neuroradiol 2003;24:1123–9.

[46] Lam WW, So NM, Wong KS, et al. B0 images obtained from diffusion-weighted echo planar sequences for the detection of intracerebral bleeds. J Neuroimaging 2003;13:99–105.

[47] Lin DD, Filippi CG, Steever AB, et al. Detection of intracranial hemorrhage: comparison between gradient-echo images and b(0) images obtained from diffusion-weighted echo-planar sequences. AJNR Am J Neuroradiol 2001;22:1275–81.

[48] Jaillard A, Hommel M, Baird AE, et al. Significance of early CT signs in acute stroke: a CT scan-diffusion MRI study. Cerebrovasc Dis 2002;13:47–56.

[49] Ozsunar Y, Grant PE, Huisman TA, et al. Evolution of water diffusion and anisotropy in hyperacute stroke: significant correlation between fractional anisotropy and T2. AJNR Am J Neuroradiol 2004;25:699–705.

[50] Russell EJ, Angtuaco EJC, Elster AD, et al. SET 42: Neuroradiology (second series) test and syllabus. Reston (VA): The American College of Radiology; 1998.

[51] Lev MH. CT versus MR for acute stroke imaging: is the "obvious" choice necessarily the correct one? AJNR Am J Neuroradiol 2003;24:1930–1.

[52] Mullins ME, Schwamm L, Maqsood M, et al. Assessment of the dense vessel sign on noncontrast head CT I: evaluation of the hyperdense middle cerebral artery sign by CTA. In: Proceedings of the American Society of Neuroradiology (ASNR) annual meeting. Oak Brook (IL): ASNR; 2004. p. 153–4.

[53] Kloska SP, Nabavi DG, Gaus C, et al. Acute stroke assessment with CT: do we need multimodal evaluation? Radiology 2004;233:79–86.

[54] Hunter GJ, Silvennoinen HM, Hamberg LM, et al. Whole-brain CT perfusion measurement of perfused cerebral blood volume in acute ischemic stroke: probability curve for regional infarction. Radiology 2003;227:725–30.

[55] Coutts SB, Lev MH, Eliasziw M, et al. ASPECTS on CTA source images versus unenhanced CT: added value in predicting final infarct extent and clinical outcome. Stroke 2004;35:2472–6.

[56] Lev MH, Farkas J, Gemmete JJ, et al. Acute stroke: improved nonenhanced CT detection–benefits of soft-copy interpretation by using variable window width and center level settings. Radiology 1999;213:150–5.

[57] Naylor AR, Rothwell PM, Bell PR. Overview of the principal results and secondary analyses from the European and North American randomised trials of endarterectomy for symptomatic carotid stenosis. Eur J Vasc Endovasc Surg 2003; 26:115–29.

[58] Koenig M, Klotz E, Luka B, et al. Perfusion CT of the brain: diagnostic approach for early detection of ischemic stroke. Radiology 1998;209:85–93.

[59] Schaefer PW, Hunter GJ, He J, et al. Predicting cerebral ischemic infarct volume with diffusion and perfusion MR imaging. AJNR Am J Neuroradiol 2002;23:1785–94.

[60] Bonaffini N, Altieri M, Rocco A, et al. Functional neuroimaging in acute stroke. Clin Exp Hypertens 2002;24:647–57.

[61] Wintermark M, Reichhart M, Cuisenaire O, et al. Comparison of admission perfusion computed tomography and qualitative diffusion- and perfusion-weighted magnetic resonance imaging in acute stroke patients. Stroke 2002;33: 2025–31.

[62] Schaefer PW, Ozsunar Y, He J, et al. Assessing tissue viability with MR diffusion and perfusion imaging. AJNR Am J Neuroradiol 2003;24: 436–43.

[63] Eastwood JD, Lev MH, Wintermark M, et al. Correlation of early dynamic CT perfusion imaging with whole-brain MR diffusion and perfusion imaging in acute hemispheric stroke. AJNR Am J Neuroradiol 2003;24:1869–75.

[64] Sanelli PC, Lev MH, Eastwood JD, et al. The effect of varying user-selected input parameters on quantitative values in CT perfusion maps. Acad Radiol 2004;11:1085–92.

[65] Goldstein LB, Jones MR, Matchar DB, et al. Improving the reliability of stroke subgroup classification using the Trial of ORG 10172 in Acute Stroke Treatment (TOAST) criteria. Stroke 2001; 32:1091–8.

[66] Kolominsky-Rabas PL, Weber M, Gefeller O, et al. Epidemiology of ischemic stroke subtypes according to TOAST criteria: incidence, recurrence, and long-term survival in ischemic stroke subtypes: a population-based study. Stroke 2001; 32:2735–40.

[67] Bryan RN, Levy LM, Whitlow WD, et al. Diagnosis of acute cerebral infarction: comparison of CT and MR imaging [see comments]. AJNR Am J Neuroradiol 1991;12:611–20.

[68] Barber PA, Darby DG, Desmond PM, et al. Identification of major ischemic change: diffusion-weighted imaging versus computed tomography. Stroke 1999;30:2059–65.

[69] Lansberg MG, Albers GW, Beaulieu C, et al. Comparison of diffusion-weighted MRI and CT in acute stroke [see comments]. Neurology 2000; 54:1557–61.

[70] Fiebach JB, Schellinger PD, Jansen O, et al. CT and diffusion-weighted MR imaging in randomized order: diffusion-weighted imaging results in higher accuracy and lower interrater variability in the diagnosis of hyperacute ischemic stroke. Stroke 2002;33:2206–10.

[71] Lovblad KO. Diffusion-weighted MRI: back to the future. Stroke 2002;33:2204–5.

[72] Mullins ME, Schaefer PW, Sorensen AG, et al. CT and conventional and diffusion-weighted MR imaging in acute stroke: study in 691 patients at presentation to the emergency department. Radiology 2002;224:353–60.

[73] Mullins ME, Cullen SP, Lev MH, et al. Acute infarct detection in a large emergency department series during the year 2000: accuracy of CT angiography (CTA). Radiology 2002;225(P):277.

[74] Beauchamp Jr NJ, Bryan RN. Acute cerebral ischemic infarction: a pathophysiologic review and radiologic perspective. AJR Am J Roentgenol 1998;171:73–84.

[75] Keir SL, Wardlaw JM. Systematic review of diffusion and perfusion imaging in acute ischemic stroke. Stroke 2000;31:2723–31.

[76] Arenillas JF, Rovira A, Molina CA, et al. Prediction of early neurological deterioration using diffusion- and perfusion-weighted imaging in hyperacute middle cerebral artery ischemic stroke. Stroke 2002;33:2197–203.

[77] Tomandl BF, Klotz E, Handschu R, et al. Comprehensive imaging of ischemic stroke with multisection CT. Radiographics 2003;23:565–92.

RADIOLOGIC
CLINICS
OF NORTH AMERICA

Radiol Clin N Am 44 (2006) 63–77

Acute Injury to the Immature Brain with Hypoxia with or Without Hypoperfusion

P. Ellen Grant, MD[a],*, David Yu, MD[b]

The most common nontraumatic mechanisms of brain injury in the neonate and young child are quite different than in the older child and adult. In this age group global brain hypoxia with or without hypoperfusion is a common mechanism of injury. Etiologies include neonatal asphyxia, choking, near drowning, sudden infant death syndrome, nonaccidental injury, severe asthma, and pneumonia. This is much different than in adults, where the most common nontraumatic brain injury is caused by focal ischemic events (from focal arterial occlusion), and when global brain hypoperfusion occurs, it is usually caused by cardiac arrest without preceding hypoxia.

When immature brain is injured because of hypoxia with or without hypoperfusion, the acute imaging findings and evolution of the imaging findings are different than the typical adult ischemic stroke. In the adult, acute ischemic stroke results in predominantly acute necrotic cell death. In the immature brain, hypoxia with or without hypoperfusion often results in a significant component of delayed cell death [1]. Although these differences may be caused in part by the different mechanisms of injury, it is also possible that programmed cell death mechanisms that are primed for the developmental process of neuronal pruning are activated more easily in the immature brain. To understand brain injury in the immature brain and the differences between the immature and mature brain, it is important to understand the possible pathways for cell death and the implications for imaging, particularly with diffusion-weighted imaging (DWI). The four major pathways for cell death are as follows [2,3]:

1. *Acute necrosis:* This occurs if there is an overwhelming insult to the cell causing unrecoverable energy failure and immediate cell death by necrosis. These injuries present as bright DWI and dark apparent diffusion coefficient (ADC) lesions (decreased ADC) within minutes. On

This article was supported by grant K23 NS42758 to Dr. Grant and in part by the National Center for Research Resources (P41RR14075) and the Mental Illness and Neuroscience Discovery (MIND) Institute.
^a Division of Pediatric Radiology, Massachusetts General Hospital, Boston, MA, USA
^b Shields MRI Health Care Group, Brockton, MA, USA
* Corresponding author. Division of Pediatric Radiology, Massachusetts General Hospital, Ellison 237, Boston, MA 02114.
E-mail address: egrant2@partners.org (P.E. Grant).

doi:10.1016/j.rcl.2005.08.001

follow-up imaging, these regions progress to volume loss with increased T2 signal caused by gliosis or cystic encephalomalacia.

2. *Delayed necrosis:* This occurs when the insult is not severe enough to cause immediate energy failure with oxygen and blood flow returning before the cell shuts down its energy mechanisms. The recovery is only transient, however, and cell death occurs by delayed necrosis. In clinical cases with histories of hypoxia or hypoperfusion and initially normal DWI studies but delayed ADC decreases, it is suspected that delayed necrosis is occurring. In these clinical scenarios, DWI abnormalities appear within hours to days of the insult. It is presumed that the ADC reductions occur for the same reasons as in immediate necrosis. Similar imaging sequelae of volume loss with gliosis or cystic encephalomalacia are expected.

3. *Delayed apoptosis:* This occurs when oxygen and blood flow return before the cell shuts down its energy mechanisms. The severity of the injury is less than with delayed necrosis because the energy metabolism recovers, but the insult is severe enough to cause the cell to undergo delayed cell death by apoptosis. To the authors' knowledge, no studies assessing the DWI signature of apoptosis have been performed because of the difficulty in developing a pure apoptotic model. This is further complicated by the fact that there are at least two different types of apoptosis: caspase dependent and caspase independent. Not only is the DWI signature unknown but there may also be more than one DWI signature for apoptosis. Given that apoptosis is a form of programmed cell death not accompanied by ATP loss and not always accompanied by sodium-potassium pump failure, it is presumed that the process of apoptosis can occur when DWI is normal. In clinical cases with progressive volume loss over weeks without an ADC decrease, it is presumed that cell death by apoptosis has occurred.

4. *Delayed aponecrosis or necroapoptosis:* This is a mixed cell death phenotype with morphologic and biochemical features of both apoptosis and necrosis that may result when apoptotic death programs are initiated and the cell energy metabolism fails, inducing necrosis; or may be a result of concomitant activation of mixed cell death mechanisms in ischemic or traumatically injured brain cells.

The primary importance of understanding these concepts of delayed cell death as an imager, is that cell death is a dynamic process with the delay in appearance of a DWI signal abnormality determined by mechanism and severity of injury and regional vulnerability. Delayed cell death is common in global brain hypoxia or hypoperfusion as blood flow and oxygen are typically restored. In these cases, the extent and severity of DWI abnormalities can change drastically over time because of variable regional vulnerability and resulting regional variations in delay to cell death. DWI within the first day can often detect the pattern of injury but is a poor predictor of the final injury. Rarely, DWI may never show significant decreases and yet long-term volume loss is observed. These scenarios are very different than the typical arterial ischemic stroke, where the lesion seen on acute DWI is very close to the final lesion volume and most cells in the DWI abnormality proceed to cell death by necrosis.

This article reviews the imaging features and evolution of immature brain injury caused by hypoxia with or without hypoperfusion in the neonate and young child. Clinical presentations and available literature on mechanisms and clinical outcomes are discussed. In many of these cases, DWI does not show the full extent of the injury but detects a pattern of injury that is important in guiding clinical care. Awareness of the delayed cell death mechanisms outlined previously is essential to understand DWI sensitivity and evolution and to provide the most accurate clinical interpretation, especially in cases of hypoxia with or without hypoperfusion.

Brain injury in the neonate

Although CT may be used acutely to rule out hemorrhage or bony fractures, MR imaging is the study of choice for assessing parenchymal brain injury in the neonate [4]. The role of MR imaging with DWI and MR spectroscopy is to provide early detection of injury (usually by day 1) [5], to determine the pattern of injury, and to assess the severity and extent of the injury. Early detection of perinatal brain injury allows the clinical team to determine if the acute brain injury is the cause of the clinical symptoms. The pattern of injury can give clues to the potential mechanisms of injury, and when combined with the severity or extent of the brain injury, this information may help manage the expectations for clinical outcome.

The imaging protocol for acute neonatal brain injury should include the following:

1. *Axial T1-weighted images:* The authors prefer axial three-dimensional spoiled gradient recalled echo with 25-degree flip angle because of its improved gray-white contrast and high

resolution. If motion is a problem, fast spin or turbo spin echo T1 images are used.

2. *Axial T2-weighted images:* The authors prefer T2-weighted fast spin or turbo spin echo because of its faster scan times, although some centers use dual echo spin echo proton density and T2-weighted sequences because of higher sensitivity to T2 change. Longer TEs improve contrast and a TE around 205 milliseconds should be used for fast spin echo T2 and 120 millisecond for spin echo T2.

3. *Axial gradient echo images:* The authors routinely perform gradient echo to detect subtle hemorrhages and venous engorgement. This is more important in centers that elect to perform fast spin or turbo spin echo over routine spin echo T2 because these are notoriously insensitive to deoxyhemoglobin and intracellular methemoglobin.

4. *Axial DWI (with calculation of ADC maps):* At pediatric centers the maximum b value used in the calculation of ADC values ranges from 700 to 1000 s/mm^2. The authors prefer a b value of 1500 s/mm^2 because of the improved contrast to noise [6]. It is helpful to have both DWI and ADC maps, because early deep gray nuclei injuries are occasionally better seen on ADC maps.

5. *MR spectroscopy of the basal ganglia and thalami and centrum semiovale on at least one side:* Longer echo times are used to assess lactate (TE of 144 or 270 milliseconds). Shorter echo times are used to assess N-acetyl aspartate (NAA) and lipid levels (TE of 35 or 144 milliseconds). Three-dimensional whole-brain sequences are preferred but time constraints and patient motion typically limit one to single voxel acquisitions.

Although fluid-attenuated inversion-recovery (FLAIR) may be useful to detect glial scarring in the chronic phase or to look for ventricular debris in acute infection, it is insensitive to acute edema in the newborn [**Fig. 1**].

Imaging should be performed as soon as clinically possible to assess for the presence and pattern of injury. In most cases, neonatal hypoxic-ischemic brain injury can be detected on DWI within 23 hours of life but the sensitivity of DWI changes over time [5,7,8]. There have been reports of negative studies in the first 24 hours [9] but often this is a moot point because most of the time the neonate is too unstable for MR imaging within 24 hours or the clinical symptoms that lead to the MR imaging occur after 24 hours. In the six neonates on whom the authors have performed DWI within 24 hours, all have been positive. Often a second MR imaging

between day 5 and 8 is helpful to rule out progression and determine the evolution of injury, because delayed white matter involvement may not be evident until this time. If transportation is difficult or scanner availability is limited, MR imaging should be performed between days 2 and 4 when DWI changes because the primary injury is easily appreciated and the pattern of injury can be identified. Although T1- and T2-weighted images often show abnormalities as early as day 1, these findings are much more subtle and DWI is essential to confirm the presence and better determine the pattern of injury. After day 8, DWI is often insensitive but in neonates presenting with perinatal encephalopathy, T1- and T2-weighted abnormalities are typically easily identified [10,11].

There are primarily three patterns of brain injury that can be identified on acute neonatal DWI, which are similar to patterns that have been described on subacute to chronic routine MR imaging:

- *Central pattern:* Involvement of the ventrolateral thalamus, corticospinal tract, or perirolandic cortex [**Fig. 2**].
- *Peripheral pattern:* Involvement of cortex and white matter but sparing of the ventrolateral thalamus, corticospinal tract, and perirolandic cortex [**Fig. 3**].
- *Focal pattern:* Vascular territory lesions [**Fig. 4**].

Central and peripheral patterns

If the global brain injury in the central and peripheral patterns is acute and severe, the neonate may present with clinical features of perinatal encephalopathy (often called hypoxic-ischemic encephalopathy). Perinatal encephalopathy is a specific clinical syndrome that requires the following criteria to be met [12]:

1. Profound metabolic or mixed acidemia (pH < 7 on umbilical cord artery blood sample if obtained).
2. One- and 5-minute Apgar scores of 0 to 3.
3. Neurologic manifestations, such as seizures, coma, or hypotonia.
4. Multisystem organ dysfunction (typically cardiovascular, gastrointestinal, renal, hematologic, or pulmonary).

When neonates meet the criteria for perinatal encephalopathy, they are more likely to have a central pattern of injury [13]. In many cases where injury is identified on DWI, however, the neonate does not meet the full criteria for perinatal encephalopathy. In fact, a neonate can have normal Apgar scores but present with seizure-like activity and have diffuse abnormalities on DWI. Perinatal encephalopathy (or hypoxic-ischemic encephalopathy) is not an imaging diagnosis and evidence

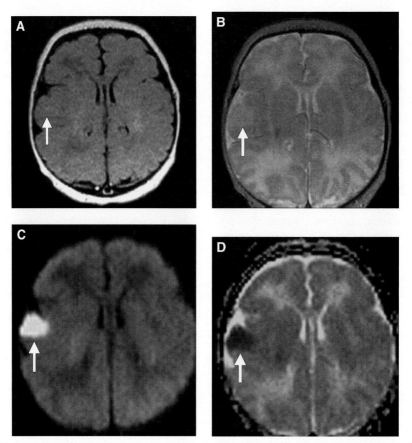

Fig. 1. Insensitivity of FLAIR. (*A*) Axial FLAIR, (*B*) T2 fast sin echo, (*C*) DWI, and (*D*) ADC map at level of bodies of lateral ventricles on day 2 of life in a term infant presenting with focal seizures. The focal vascular territory ischemic injury that is easily identified on DWI and ADC images (*arrow*) is not seen on the FLAIR image (*arrow*), but is visible on the T2 fast spin echo image (*arrow*).

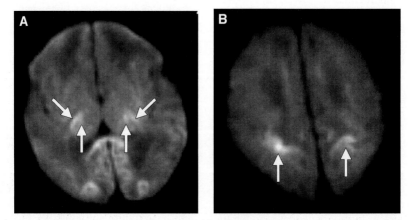

Fig. 2. Central pattern of DWI injury. Bright DWI signal involves (*A*) the posterior limb internal capsule (*angled arrows*), the ventrolateral thalamus (*vertical arrows*), and (*B*) the perirolandic cortex (*arrows*). The margins of the DWI lesions are often indistinct.

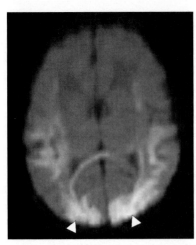

Fig. 3. Peripheral pattern of DWI injury. Bright DWI signal involves diffuse regions of white matter and cortex (*arrowheads*). The margins of the DWI bright lesions are often indistinct.

of brain injury may be present on MR imaging in the absence of clinical perinatal encephalopathy.

Neonatal hypoxic-ischemic injury is associated with many risk factors. Antepartum associations include maternal hypotension, infertility treatment, and thyroid disease. Intrapartum associations include forceps delivery, breech extraction, cord prolapse, abruptio placentae, and maternal fever. Postpartum risks include severe respiratory distress, sepsis, and shock [14].

The central pattern is thought to result when there is global profound lack of oxygen and blood flow (hypoxia and ischemia) to the brain for a relatively short period of time (minutes) resulting in injury of regions of high energy demand [1]. Pathologic studies of term neonates who succumbed to a profound hypoxic ischemic event show relative cortical sparing and deep gray matter injury particularly involving hippocampi, lateral geniculate nuclei, putamen, ventrolateral thalami, and dorsal mesencephalon. These regions have high concentrations of excitatory amino acids (glutamate, aspartate) and corresponding N-methyl-D-aspartate receptors. Excessive uptake of excitatory amino acids by N-methyl-D-aspartate receptors results in depolarization of neuronal membranes, excessive calcium influx, activation of second messenger systems, mobilization of internal calcium stores, activation of lipases and proteases, generation of free fatty acids and free radicals, mitochondrial dysfunction, depletion of energy stores, and ultimate neuronal death. Mature deep gray nuclei also contain myelin and are also undergoing active myelination with high-energy requirements at term. The combination of increased excitatory amino acids and N-methyl-D-aspartate receptors and active myelina-

tion may cause these regions to be more susceptible to injury following profound asphyxia [11].

Profound asphyxia before 32 weeks gestational age results in injury to thalami, basal ganglia, and brainstem. Compared with profound asphyxia in term infants, perirolandic cortex is spared. Thalamic involvement is similar but basal ganglia involvement is less, with decreased scarring. Basal ganglia begin to myelinate at 33 to 35 weeks gestational age compared with thalami at 23 to 25 weeks. Barkovich and Sargent [10] speculate that the higher energy demands from active myelination within the thalami but not the basal ganglia before 32 weeks account for the increased susceptibility of the thalamus to profound asphyxia at this gestational age. In addition, the basal ganglia, which have a lower white matter content and delayed onset of myelination compared with thalami, may suffer less injury and develop less scarring because of presence of fewer cells that are able to mount an astroglial response. Without an astroglial response, brain reacts to injury by resorption resulting in volume loss and cavitation, which is seen in the basal ganglia.

The peripheral pattern is thought to result from a global brain hypoxia and ischemia that is more prolonged (hours) but less profound and is often termed *partial asphyxia* [10,13,15]. This pattern of injury primarily involves cortex and white matter that is not actively myelinating. It is thought that the immature white matter is more vulnerable to ischemia-related injury than mature white matter. In particular, preoligodendrocytes and oligodendrocyte progenitor cells are more susceptible to antioxidant depletion and free radical exposure than mature oligodendrocytes. Oligodendrocyte

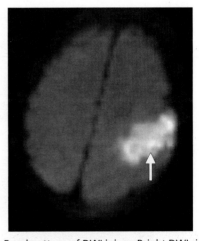

Fig. 4. Focal pattern of DWI injury. Bright DWI signal is seen in a focal region corresponding to an arterial vascular territory. Typically, the margins of the DWI bright lesion are sharp (*arrow*).

progenitor cells express glutamate receptors including α-amino-3-hydroxy-5-methyl-4-isoxazole propionic acid (AMPA) and kainite receptors making them vulnerable to excess activation by glutamatergic neurotransmission and cell death by excitotoxicity [14].

There is variation in the peripheral pattern depending on gestational age that is thought to depend on the maturation of the brain and vascular supply at time of insult. In premature neonates, periventricular white matter is supplied by ventriculopetal arteries coursing inward from the cerebral cortex. With maturity, ventriculofugal arteries develop coursing peripherally from the ventricular wall. Ventriculofugal arteries develop between 32 and 44 weeks gestational age. Development of ventriculofugal arteries is believed to shift the watershed region in neonates from periventricular at earlier ages to cortical at term, explaining the centrifugal shift of injury with brain maturity. In the immature nervous system, damaged tissue undergoes liquefaction necrosis and is resorbed. Repair process with astrocyte mitosis and growth is believed to begin developing only at 28 weeks, explaining why earlier injury is not accompanied by gliosis [16]. Although the changing watershed zone may play a significant role in this pattern of injury, more recently a role for inflammatory mediators and altered innate immunity has been postulated [17]. The authors have also begun to question if hypoxia may play a larger role than hypoperfusion. The physiologic mechanisms behind these types of injury are not completely understood.

DWI abnormalities in central patterns of injury caused by profound insults may underestimate the degree of injury on follow-up but typically brainstem involvement on acute DWI or markedly decreased ADCs in the posterior limb internal capsule portend a poorer prognosis [**Fig. 5**] [18,19]. Subtle diffuse increased T2 signal and bright T1 signal can often be seen in the putamen and thalami by 2 days [20]. By 6 or 7 days decreased T2 signal is often seen in the putamen and thalami. The T1 changes become more focal by about 8 to 10 days [20].

In peripheral patterns of injury, regions of bright DWI signal and decreased ADC involve both white matter and cortex [see **Fig. 3**]. Often loss of gray-white distinction can be seen by 2 days on T2-weighted images in areas with cortical involvement but T2 images underestimate the extent of white matter involvement. Follow-up imaging studies show a spectrum of outcomes with the T2- and T1-weighted abnormalities often involving a smaller region than the initial DWI abnormality [**Fig. 6**]. Reports of preterm infants suggest that the DWI abnormalities primarily involve the white matter in infants less than 36 weeks [7].

Because of the difficulties in predicting tissue outcome based on DWI and ADC maps at any one point in time, the authors avoid the term "stroke" or "infarct" when describing these lesions to the neonatal intensive care team. These terms imply that the area with bright DWI signal and low ADC is irreversibly injured with all cell types in the abnormal region undergoing necrosis. The authors have adopted the term "metabolic stress or insult" to imply that the tissue with the abnormal DWI signal has experienced a severe enough insult to at least alter its energy metabolism and to allow for the possibility that some or all of the cellular ele-

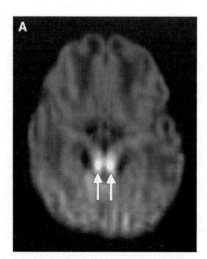
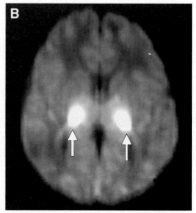

Fig. 5. Central pattern with brainstem involvement. Bright DWI signal (*A*) in the posterior brainstem (*arrows*) and (*B*) in the ventrolateral thalamus (*arrows*) on day 1 in a neonate that died within 1 week after presenting with Apgar scores of 0, 0, and 0 at 1, 5, and 10 minutes, respectively.

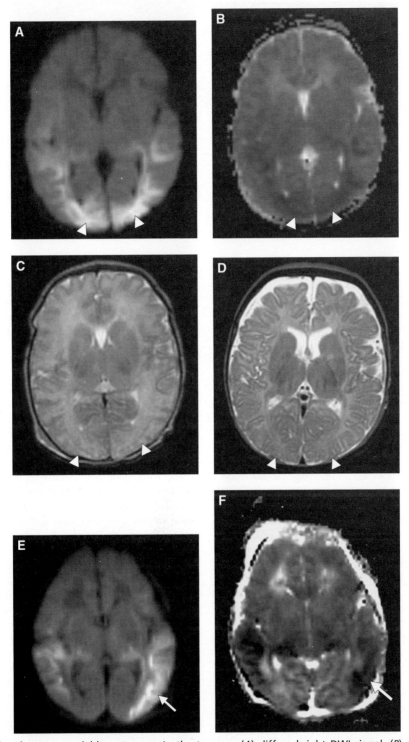

Fig. 6. Peripheral pattern variable outcomes. In the top row (A) diffuse bright DWI signal, (B) corresponding decreased ADC, and (C) increased T2 in the cortical gray matter on day 2 (*arrowheads*) results in (D) mild diffuse volume loss and a smaller region of subtle ulegyria in the occipital regions on T2 4 months later. (E) Bilateral but asymmetric DWI signal worse on the left (*arrow*), (F) corresponding to decreased ADC, slightly more extensive on the left (*arrow*), and (G) associated with loss of gray-white distinction on the left (*arrow*) progresses to (H) more extensive volume loss on T2 (*arrow*) 4 months later.

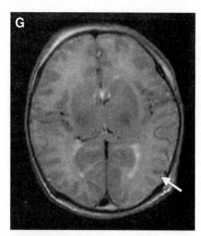
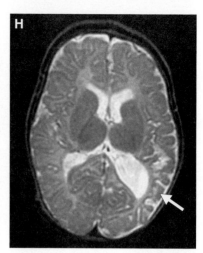

Fig. 6 (continued).

ments may recover and that selective cellular death may occur instead of full-thickness injury.

Lactate is often identified in the basal ganglia and thalamic region in encephalopathic neonates and may be helpful in short-term prognosis [21,22]. The role of MR spectroscopy in neonates that are not encephalopathic and in preterm infants is less clear. When present in the acute stage it suggests that mitochondrial function has been impaired and anaerobic metabolism is occurring. Because of the frequent association of hypoxic-ischemic brain injury with rebound hyperperfusion, the absence of lactate does not exclude anaerobic metabolism because the authors have found that rebound hyperperfusion can decrease tissue lactate levels.

Unlike in adult ischemic stroke, in neonatal hypoxic-ischemic injury, reperfusion occurs before the cells begin to undergo immediate necrosis. In immediate necrosis, failure of ATP production and glutamate-mediated toxicity result in influx of sodium and calcium with cellular edema and rupture. This is the typical result of ischemic infarction in adults. In neonates suffering from hypoxic-ischemic injury reperfusion occurs and if the mitochondria have not been irreversibly injured, the cells can once again produce ATP. In this context, cell death is not necessarily averted but cell death pathways may be converted from immediate necrosis to delayed cell death by either necrosis, apoptosis, or a combination of both [2,3]. This explains the delayed nadir in ADCs and the appearance of new areas of decreased ADC seen in the first few days after an insult that has been reported [8,9,19,23,24].

Currently, there is still little information on the correlation between MR imaging findings in the first week of life and outcome at school age when the full impact on neuropsychologic function be-

gins to become apparent. Outcome studies based on entrance criteria of perinatal distress are applicable only to that population. The outcome for neonates presenting with DWI abnormalities in the absence of perinatal distress cannot be determined from these studies.

Focal pattern

Arterial strokes are most common in term infants. Risk factors include history of infertility, pre-eclampsia, prolonged rupture of membranes, and chorioamnionitis with marked increases when multiple risk factors are present [25].

The focal pattern is caused by focal arterial occlusions. In most cases the cause is unknown, but possibilities include emboli, thrombosis, or transient spasm. Typically, these are focal events on an otherwise normal brain with no evidence of global brain involvement [26,27]. As expected, most of these neonates are not encephalopathic and typically present within the first few days of life not with focal neurologic deficits but with a focal seizure. The typical history is a newborn with normal delivery and normal Apgar scores presenting with focal seizure activity around day 2 of life. Although it is commonly thought that these injuries occur at or around the time of birth, the reasons for the delay in overt seizure activity are unclear.

In the few cases the authors have studied with perfusion imaging, hyperperfusion when imaged on day 2 is commonly seen. In addition, preliminary data suggest that the region of tissue with T2 abnormalities on follow-up may be slightly smaller than the initial DWI abnormality, consistent with these injuries reperfusing more rapidly than is typical for adult strokes and delayed mechanisms of cell death may play a larger role. The role of apoptosis in neonatal stroke has been also supported by animal models [28].

Outcomes are typically quite good in these lesions compared with the diffuse injuries. Concomitant involvement of basal ganglia, corpus callosum, and posterior limb of the internal capsule has been reported to predict the development of hemiparesis, with no child with one or two of these structures involved developing hemiparesis [29].

Brain injury in the young child

Drowning, choking, and nonaccidental trauma are among the most common forms of brain injury in the young child. In near drowning and choking and often in nonaccidental trauma, hypoxic hypoxia occurs followed by reoxygenation when resuscitated. If the hypoxia is prolonged, cardiac dysfunction or arrest may occur, resulting in a period of decreased or absent perfusion and hypoxia. With resuscitation, reoxygenation and reperfusion occur. MR imaging plays an important role in the assessment of cerebral injury because often the child is sedated in the field, limiting the clinical examination on arrival to the emergency room, or the history is not forthcoming.

When imaging in the young child exposed to a hypoxic or anoxic event with or without associated cardiac arrest the authors recommend that the protocol include the following sequences:

1. Axial T1-weighted
2. Axial T2-weighted fast spin echo
3. Axial DWI
4. MR spectroscopy with TE of 35 or 144 ms, including the lentiform nucleus and occipital cortex
5. Perfusion (optional)

At the authors' institution, imaging is preformed at the earliest feasible time to assess for the presence or absence of injury and to detect the pattern and severity of the injury. If normal, a second study at approximately 48 hours is performed to determine if there is delayed injury. When transportation is difficult, imaging between 2 and 4 days is likely most helpful for diagnosis of injury and for prognosis.

Anoxia and hypoperfusion

In children following asphyxia (anoxia) and subsequent cardiorespiratory arrest, those who have vegetative outcomes or succumb to the injury typically have abnormal MR imaging with DWI and MR spectroscopy within the first 12 to 24 hours. The actual time at which the imaging becomes abnormal is not well documented but it probably depends on the severity of the insult, with most severe anoxic hypoperfusion injuries becoming abnormal within 12 hours [**Fig. 7**]. The initial abnormalities are bright DWI low ADC in the posterior lateral lentiform and ventrolateral thalamus (as in the neonate) within approximately 12 to 24 hours, which precede T1 and T2 signal changes. If dynamic susceptibility contrast perfusion-weighted MR imaging is performed at this time, the authors have noted marked increases in relative cerebral blood volume in these regions of decreased ADC indicating rebound hyperperfusion in this area. Unlike neonatal profound hypoxia and hypoperfusion with reperfusion and unlike the deep gray injury in most adult cases of cardiac arrest, however, the injury shows significant progression over time. By approximately 48 hours, the entire basal ganglia and thalamus become involved and the perirolandic and visual cortex [see **Fig. 7**], with MR spectroscopy in DWI-abnormal cortical areas showing elevated lactate and glutamate. Between 48 and 72 hours, the entire cortex becomes involved and diffuse cerebral swelling is evident. White matter ADCs decrease and cortical ADCs normalize. Abnormalities on routine MR imaging sequences and MR spectroscopy by day 2 portents a poor prognosis but a normal study cannot rule out injury until day 3 or 4. Best correlation for MR imaging and MR spectroscopy findings with outcome was at 3 to 4 days with 100% positive and negative predictive value for poor outcome [30]. The predictive values of DWI and perfusion have not been determined, but in the authors' experience [31], DWI abnormalities within 12 to 24 hours have a poor prognosis. A similar progression with time has also been documented on CT, although the detection of the initial findings does not occur until after 24 hours, and on MR imaging with MR spectroscopy [16,30]. At 4 to 6 days, hemorrhage may develop within the basal ganglia or cortex. MR imaging with DWI shows massive cerebral swelling; normalization of cortical ADCs (likely caused by vasogenic edema); and marked white matter ADC decreases. MR spectroscopy shows significant loss of all metabolites in the cortex and lactate. In some cases where mannitol has been given, mannitol may be detected as a peak at 3.9 ppm [**Fig. 8**].

Hypoxia-anoxia with maintained perfusion

For short durations, isolated hypoxia or anoxia without ischemia is better tolerated both clinically and pathologically. With isolated hypoxia there is preservation of cerebral blood flow allowing continued supply of nutrients and removal of toxic products [32]. In cases with respiratory arrest that do not progress to cardiac arrest, the cerebral injury is primarily caused by hypoxic hypoxia with reoxygenation during recovery or resuscitation.

Imaging findings with isolated hypoxic hypoxia are not well documented, with most studies focusing on ischemic hypoxia. In the authors' (albeit limited) experience, it seems that delayed injury with selective involvement of the white matter (postanoxic leukoencephalopathy) may be underappreciated. In the authors' cases, respiratory arrest was documented or significant respiratory compromise was highly suspected but no cardiac arrest or dysfunction occurred. In the literature, similar inju-

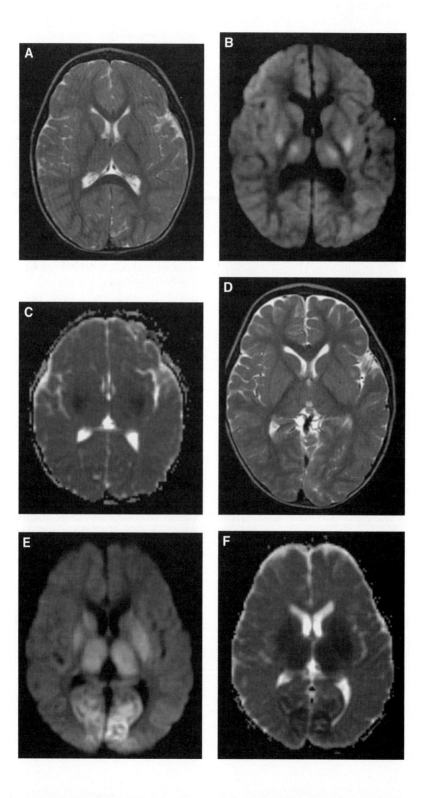

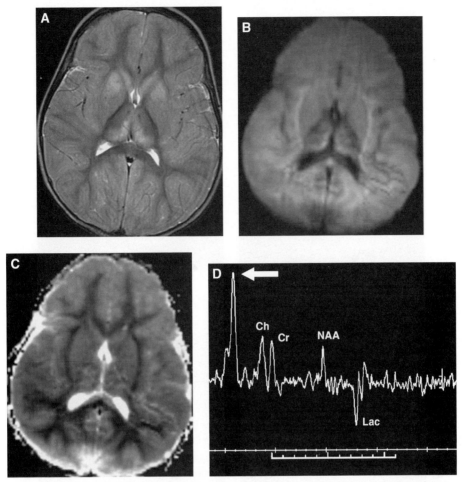

Fig. 8. Severe anoxia and hypoperfusion. Four days after cardiorespiratory arrest caused by near drowning in another toddler, (*A*) the T2 fast spin echo shows diffuse cerebral swelling with increased T2 in gray matter. (*B*) DWI shows increased signal throughout the brain. (*C*) On the ADC map the gray matter ADCs are close to normal but the white matter ADCs are markedly reduced. (*D*) MR spectroscopy in the parietal lobe gray matter shows markedly reduced choline (Ch), creatine (Cr), and NAA peaks indicating profound tissue injury, the presence of lactate (Lac) indicating anaerobic metabolism, and an unusual peak of 3.9 ppm corresponding to mannitol (*arrow*).

ries can be seen in adults with respiratory arrest, carbon dioxide poisoning, cyanide poisoning, cardiac arrest, or drug overdose [33]. Initial MR imaging with DWI and MR spectroscopy is typically normal but by approximately day 2 (in the adult literature it may be many days later), marked ADC decreases throughout the white matter are noted [Fig. 9] [31]. These injuries evolve to diffuse

volume loss often with abnormally increased T2 on long-term follow-up.

Because these children are so young, clinical evidence of the diffuse white matter injury is often not obvious. Without imaging identification of the white matter injury that becomes apparent approximately 2 days after the insult, significant risk to cognitive function may not have

Fig. 7. Severe anoxia and hypoperfusion. (*A*) Eighteen hours after cardiorespiratory arrest secondary to choking the T2 fast spin echo shows no abnormality but (*B*) DWI shows abnormally bright signal in the posterior putamen and ventrolateral thalamus. (*C*) The corresponding ADC map shows that the DWI bright regions have decreased ADC. Two days after cardiorespiratory arrest in the same toddler, (*D*) only subtle increased T2 signal is noted in the basal ganglia, thalami, and occipital cortex on T2 fast spin echo, whereas (*E*) the DWI shows marked increased signal in these regions and in the perirolandic cortex (not shown). (*F*) These areas correspond to regions of decreased ADC on the ADC map. The cause of the brain volume loss between (*A*) and (*D*) is unknown but is likely caused by mannitol and other medical interventions.

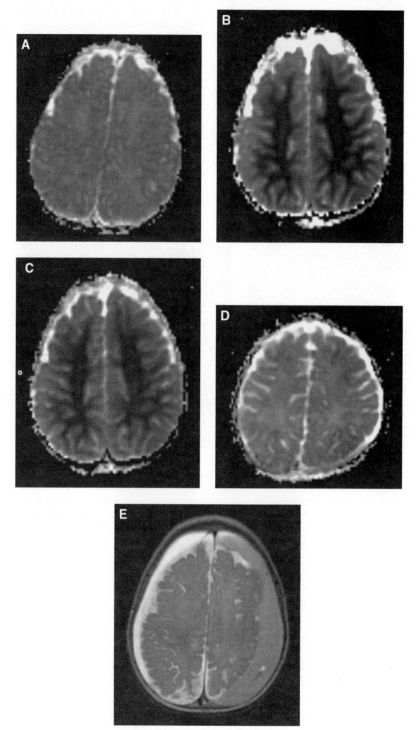

Fig. 9. Hypoxia with delayed white matter injury. Progression of injury on ADC maps with (*A*) normal ADC at 18 hours, (*B*) maximal white matter ADC decrease at 2 days, (*C*) less marked but persistent white matter ADC decrease at 4 days, (*D*) elevation of white matter ADCs at 8 days, and (*E*) an axial T2-weighted image showing marked volume loss 2 months after event with secondary bilateral subdural collections.

been identified and early intervention may not have occurred.

Limitations of diffusion-weighted imaging

As a result of the authors' experience in the adult stroke population, where cell death occurs predominantly by acute necrosis, it is common to assume that the DWI obtained during the acute phase represents the full extent of the cerebral injury. If normal, an acute injury is ruled out. Although a normal DWI rules out acute necrosis, it does not rule out activation of delayed cell death pathways. Unlike in the adult, in the infant and young child cerebral insults associated with hypoxia with or without hypoperfusion followed by reoxygenation with or without reperfusion commonly occur. The immature brain has primed delayed (or pro-

grammed) cell death pathways used for normal processes of neuronal pruning that can become overactivated after an insult. In addition, the reoxygenation and reperfusion results in restored energy supply, which may avert acute necrotic cell death in favor of delayed apoptosis, necrosis, or mixed cell death. A normal DWI in the acute setting or regions with normal DWI signal in the acute setting does not rule out significant injury and impending cell death. In fact, in one example, despite the presence of an acute cerebellar reversal sign on CT (suggesting an anoxic insult), multiple DWI studies in the first week were normal with only a minimal decline in the ADCs in the right visual cortex on day two. On follow-up imaging, diffuse cerebral volume loss was noted [Fig. 10] [31]. This case suggests that volume loss, suggestive

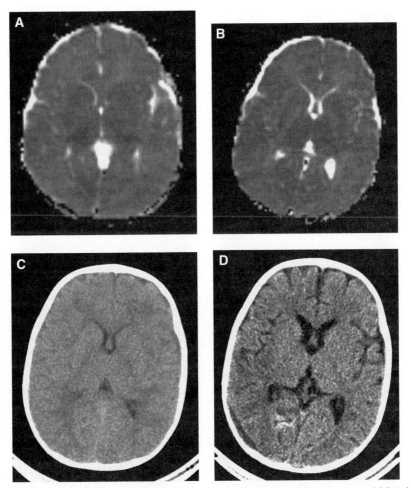

Fig. 10. Cerebral volume loss with no acute DWI abnormality. ADC maps at (*A*) 12 hours and (*B*) 3 days compared with (*C*) CT before cerebral insult and (*D*) CT 18 days after the insult. Despite near normal ADC maps, interval volume loss can be seen by comparing CT scans, where the study 18 days after the insult (*D*) shows not only a small region of increased attenuation likely representing early calcification in the right visual cortex but also diffuse volume loss despite lack of diffuse ADC changes.

of apoptotic cell death, may occur in the absence of significant ADC decreases.

Summary

Hypoxia with or without hypoperfusion is a common mechanism of injury in the immature brain and can result in normal or minimally abnormal imaging studies in the first 12 hours. Often, injury progresses over time suggesting a central role for delayed cell death pathways. An awareness of the patterns of injury associated with different mechanisms of injury and the central role of delayed cell death pathways in injury evolution is important for the radiologist to understand the significance and potential outcome of these injuries.

References

[1] Johnston MV, Trescher WH, Ishida A, et al. Neurobiology of hypoxic-ischemic injury in the developing brain. Pediatr Res 2001;49:735–41.

[2] Leist M, Jaattela M. Four deaths and a funeral: from caspases to alternative mechanisms. Nat Rev Mol Cell Biol 2001;2:589–98.

[3] Yakovlev AG, Faden AI. Mechanisms of neural cell death: implications for development of neuroprotective treatment strategies. Neurorx 2004;1:5–16.

[4] Ment LR, Bada HS, Barnes P, et al. Practice parameter: neuroimaging of the neonate: report of the Quality Standards Subcommittee of the American Academy of Neurology and the Practice Committee of the Child Neurology Society. Neurology 2002;58:1726–38.

[5] Barkovich AJ, Westmark KD, Bedi HS, et al. Proton spectroscopy and diffusion imaging on the first day of life after perinatal asphyxia: preliminary report. AJNR Am J Neuroradiol 2001; 22:1786–94.

[6] Pectasides M, Pienaar R, Matsuda KM, et al. Optimizing diffusion weighted imaging in neonatal vascular territory injuries. Presented at the International Society for Magnetic Resonance in Medicine 13th Annual Scientific Meeting and Exhibition. Miami Beach, Florida, May 7–13, 2005.

[7] Inder T, Huppi PS, Zientara GP, et al. Early detection of periventricular leukomalacia by diffusion-weighted magnetic resonance imaging techniques. J Pediatr 1999;134:631–4.

[8] Takeoka M, Soman TB, Yoshii A, et al. Diffusion-weighted images in neonatal cerebral hypoxic-ischemic injury. Pediatr Neurol 2002;26:274–81.

[9] Robertson RL, Ben-Sira L, Barnes PD, et al. MR line-scan diffusion-weighted imaging of term neonates with perinatal brain ischemia. AJNR Am J Neuroradiol 1999;20:1658–70.

[10] Barkovich AJ, Sargent SK. Profound asphyxia in the premature infant: imaging findings. AJNR Am J Neuroradiol 1995;16:1837–46.

[11] Barkovich AJ. MR and CT evaluation of profound neonatal and infantile asphyxia. AJNR Am J Neuroradiol 1992;13(3):959–72 [discussion 973–5].

[12] The American College of Obstetricians and Gynecologists' Task Force on Neonatal Encephalopathy and Cerebral Palsy and the American College of Obstetricians and Gynecologists and the American Academy of Pediatrics: criteria required to define an acute intrapartum hypoxic event as sufficient to cause cerebral palsy. In: Neonatal encephalopathy and cerebral palsy: defining the pathogenesis and pathophysiology. Washington DC: American College of Obstetricians and Gynecologists; 2003. p. 74–80.

[13] Sie LT, van der Knaap MS, Oosting J, et al. MR patterns of hypoxic-ischemic brain damage after prenatal, perinatal or postnatal asphyxia. Neuropediatrics 2000;31:128–36.

[14] Ferriero DM. Neonatal brain injury. N Engl J Med 2004;351:1985–95.

[15] Barkovich AJ, Truwit CL. Brain damage from perinatal asphyxia: correlation of MR findings with gestational age. AJNR Am J Neuroradiol 1990;11:1087–96.

[16] Barkovich A. Pediatric neuroimaging. 3rd edition. Philadelphia: Lippincott, Williams & Wilkins; 2000.

[17] Lassiter HA. The role of complement in neonatal hypoxic-ischemic cerebral injury. Clin Perinatol 2004;31:117–27.

[18] Hunt RW, Neil JJ, Coleman LT, et al. Apparent diffusion coefficient in the posterior limb of the internal capsule predicts outcome after perinatal asphyxia. Pediatrics 2004;114:999–1003.

[19] Wolf RL, Zimmerman RA, Clancy R, et al. Quantitative apparent diffusion coefficient measurements in term neonates for early detection of hypoxic-ischemic brain injury: initial experience. Radiology 2001;218:825–33.

[20] Barkovich AJ, Westmark K, Partridge C, et al. Perinatal asphyxia: MR findings in the first 10 days. AJNR Am J Neuroradiol 1995;16:427–38.

[21] Barkovich AJ, Baranski K, Vigneron D, et al. Proton MR spectroscopy for the evaluation of brain injury in asphyxiated, term neonates. AJNR Am J Neuroradiol 1999;20:1399–405.

[22] Kadri M, Shu S, Holshouser B, et al. Proton magnetic resonance spectroscopy improves outcome prediction in perinatal CNS insults. J Perinatol 2003;23:181–5.

[23] McKinstry RC, Miller JH, Snyder AZ, et al. A prospective, longitudinal diffusion tensor imaging study of brain injury in newborns. Neurology 2002;59:824–33.

[24] Soul JS, Robertson RL, Tzika AA, et al. Time course of changes in diffusion-weighted magnetic resonance imaging in a case of neonatal encephalopathy with defined onset and duration of hypoxic-ischemic insult. Pediatrics 2001;108: 1211–4.

[25] Lee J, Croen LA, Backstrand KH, et al. Maternal and infant characteristics associated with perina-

tal arterial stroke in the infant. JAMA 2005;293: 723–9.

[26] Matsuda KM, Krishnamoorthy KS, Grant PE. ADC changes in neonatal brain injury and outcome. In: 48th Annual Society of Pediatric Radiology, May 3–7, 2005. New Orleans (LA): Springer; 2005. p. S70–1.

[27] Matsuda KM, Lopez CJ, Pectasides M, et al. Apparent diffusion coefficients (ADC) in neonatal brain injury: patterns of injury and outcome. Presented at the American Society of Neuroradiology 43rd Annual Meeting. Toronto, Canada, May 23–27, 2005.

[28] Manabat C, Han BH, Wendland M, et al. Reperfusion differentially induces caspase-3 activation in ischemic core and penumbra after stroke in immature brain. Stroke 2003;34:207–13.

[29] Boardman JP, Ganesan V, Rutherford MA, et al. Magnetic resonance image correlates of hemipa-

resis after neonatal and childhood middle cerebral artery stroke. Pediatrics 2005;115:321–6.

[30] Dubowitz DJ, Bluml S, Arcinue E, et al. MR of hypoxic encephalopathy in children after near drowning: correlation with quantitative proton MR spectroscopy and clinical outcome. AJNR Am J Neuroradiol 1998;19:1617–27.

[31] Pectasides M, Buckley AW, Krishnamoorthy KS, et al. Respiratory ± cardiac arrest: delayed ADC decreases. In: 48th Annual Society of Pediatric Radiology, May 3–7, 2005. New Orleans (LA): Springer; 2005. p. S72.

[32] Singhal AB, Topcuoglu MA, Koroshetz WJ. Diffusion MRI in three types of anoxic encephalopathy. J Neurol Sci 2002;196:37–40.

[33] Chalela JA, Wolf RL, Maldjian JA, et al. MRI identification of early white matter injury in anoxic-ischemic encephalopathy. Neurology 2001;56: 481–5.

ELSEVIER
SAUNDERS

Update on Multiple Sclerosis

Jack H. Simon, MD, PhD*

Immediately after the first descriptions of the application of MR imaging to multiple sclerosis (MS) in the early 1980s, MR imaging assumed an important role beyond that of CT in increasing confidence in the diagnosis, and in excluding clinical presentations mimicking MS but caused by other pathology. In large part because MR imaging could provide multiple important outcome measures in MS clinical trials, a great deal of information was collected from these and related studies relevant to the natural history of MS lesions, the underlying pathology, the sensitivity of MR imaging to pathology in the normal-appearing tissues, and its value as a predictor of clinical MS. Recently, MR imaging has provided new tools that can be used to understand the relationship between the

focal and diffuse pathology, including the quantitative MR imaging techniques (magnetization transfer, T1 and T2 relaxation based methods, diffusion tensor MR imaging and tractography, MR spectroscopy, perfusion), and the functional consequences and early compensatory mechanisms that the central nervous system (CNS) uses to minimize disability based on functional MR imaging studies.

In this update on MS, the basic features of the focal MR imaging lesions and the underlying pathology are first reviewed, including new insights into MS as a disease with early axonal pathology. Next, the diffuse pathology in the normal-appearing white matter (NAWM) and normal-appearing gray matter (NAGM) as revealed by conventional and quantitative MR imaging techniques is discussed,

Department of Radiology, University of Colorado Health Sciences Center, Denver, CO, USA
* Department of Radiology, University of Colorado Health Sciences Center, 4200 East Ninth Avenue, Box A-034, Denver, CO 80262.
E-mail address: jack.simon@uchsc.edu

doi:10.1016/j.rcl.2005.08.005

including reference to how the focal and diffuse pathology may be in part linked through axonal-neuronal degeneration. MR imaging findings have been shown to be predictive of MS, and the MR imaging criteria incorporated for the first time into formal clinical diagnostic criteria for MS are next discussed. Finally, a discussion is provided as to how MR imaging is used in monitoring subclinical disease either before or subsequent to initiation of treatment, in identifying aggressive subclinical disease, and treatment of nonresponders.

Clinical multiple sclerosis overview

MS is a chronic, inflammatory, demyelinating disease of the CNS that has been estimated to affect about 250,000 to 350,000 individuals in the United States and more than 2.5 million worldwide. The etiology remains unknown, although environmental (viral) and immune-mediated factors in genetically susceptible individuals are thought to be responsible. Typically beginning in early adulthood, the prognosis is highly variable, but left untreated 50% of patients require assistance in walking within 15 years of onset, and more than 50% have cognitive deficits detected by formal neuropsychologic testing, many in the early relapsing stages of disease [1,2].

Approximately 80% to 85% of patients present with a relapsing-remitting course, with symptoms and signs evolving over days, and typically improving over weeks. The female/male ratio is about 2:1 for relapsing MS. A secondary progressive course develops after about 10 years in as many as 50% of patients, with disease progression occurring between relapses, and relapses less frequent over time. In about 15% of patients, the disease is progressive from onset (primary progressive MS), with males and females more equally affected. Rarely, patients show an initially progressive course with subsequent superimposed relapses (progressive-relapsing MS) [3]. About 10% to 20% of MS patients do well for 20 years, and are considered to have "benign" MS, a diagnosis that can at this time only be made in retrospect [4], and included in this group may be individuals with unrecognized cognitive deficits.

Presenting signs and symptoms of MS frequently include those associated with a clinically isolated syndrome (CIS) affecting one optic nerve (optic neuritis); brainstem or cerebellum (diplopia-internuclear ophthalmoplegia, ataxia, trigeminal neuralgia); or a spinal cord syndrome with partial transverse myelitis (weakness, numbness). Bladder-bowel symptoms are common. Fatigue is described by many patients as especially debilitating [1,2].

Relapsing MS is a treatable disease [1,2]. Therapy for MS is based on immunomodulatory agents including interferon beta-1a, interferon beta-1b, and glatiramer acetate. In late 2004 the Food and Drug Administration approved a monoclonal antibody (anti-α_4 integrin) that inhibits the trafficking of leukocytes across the CNS endothelium by blocking binding of $\alpha_4\beta_1$ integrin to a vascular cell adhesion molecule [5], but natalizumab (Tysabri) was voluntarily suspended from the market based on safety concerns as progressive multifocal leucoencephalopathy (PML) was discovered with an occurrence greater than expected as it occurred in a few trial patients on combination therapy. The effectiveness of immunomodulatory or other therapies is more difficult to demonstrate in secondary progressive MS, in part because these treatments probably do not target already injured tissue. Betaseron and mitoxantrone are approved for treatment of secondary progressive MS. There are no proved therapies for primary progressive MS [1]. MR imaging–based outcome measures have been instrumental in the approval process for the MS therapies. The cumulative number of gadolinium-enhancing lesions on monthly MR imaging is the primary outcome measure for many phase II trials [6]. Enhancing lesions, number of new and enlarging T2 lesions, and T2 lesion volume change are important secondary outcome measures in phase III (definitive) trials [6,7].

The focal and diffuse multiple sclerosis pathology by MR imaging

The MS pathology detected by direct neuropathologic examination or MR imaging is both focal and diffuse. Focal, classic MS lesions represent a range of pathology from nondestructive edema to injury from demyelination and most severe injury related to axonal loss [8]. The diffuse pathology may be evident by MR imaging only indirectly as indicated by atrophy [9–11], or detected in the normal-appearing white or gray matter by the advanced quantitative MR imaging methodologies [12,13]. As discussed later, there is mounting evidence that the clinical and cognitive consequences of the MS pathology require an understanding of the focal pathology, yet the diffuse pathology may be equally if not more important.

Enhancing lesions, the blood-brain barrier, and inflammation

The acute enhancing MS lesion, which is almost always associated with hyperintensity on T2-weighted imaging, is visualized as a result of abnormal leakage and accumulation of contrast material across disrupted tight junctions of the vas-

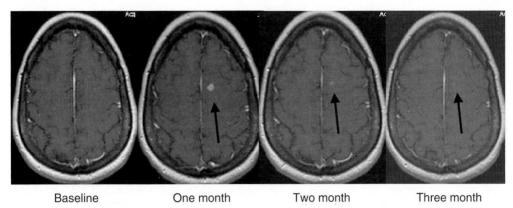

Baseline	One month	Two month	Three month

Fig. 1. Time course for enhancing lesion. Serial monthly MR imaging shows development of a new enhancing lesion (*arrows*) at 1 month, and the typical decrease in size over the subsequent 2 months. The duration of enhancement can range from less than 1 week to about 16 weeks. The time course for enhancement in MS parallels that for inflammation, but more accurately enhancement measures the integrity of the blood-brain barrier.

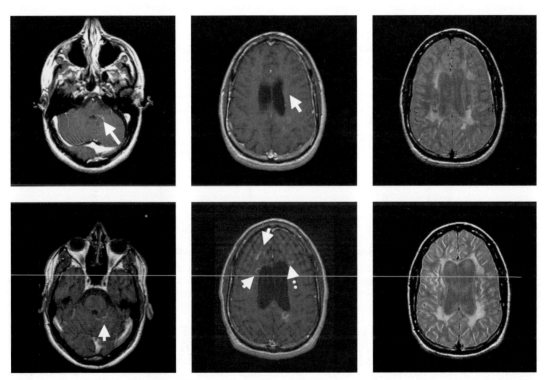

Fig. 2. Aggressive MS over 2 years. Patient with relatively early disease onset at age 15 and death 7 years later related to MS. Disease was initially relapsing-remitting but converted relatively quickly to secondary progressive MS (progression without relapses). Top row: contrast-enhancement left pons (*left*) and left frontal-parietal white matter (*middle*) both showing a relatively rare edge enhancement pattern (*arrows*). Typical confluent T2 hyperintensities and mild-moderate volume loss based on lateral ventricle size (*right*). Bottom row: two years later MR imaging shows different edge enhancing lesions (*arrows*) in posterior fossa (*left*) and both edge enhancement (*arrows*) and ring enhancement (*dotted arrow*) in deep white matter along the lateral ventricles (*middle*). Progressive volume loss based on moderately large lateral ventricles and more extensive confluent T2 hyperintensity (*right*). This enhancement pattern is relatively rare (*arrows*), and in this case apparently related to an aggressive disease course. Ring enhancement has also been associated with more severe pathology, but not all patients with ring enhancement show an aggressive course by MR imaging.

cular endothelium that are a crucial component of the blood-brain barrier [14]. The factors associated with the initial barrier disruption are complex, but central to this process is entrance of activated T cells through the junctions of the capillary endothelium. These activated lymphocytes recognize CNS antigen and trigger a cytokine-chemokine cascade that further mediates disruption of the blood-brain barrier [15,16] with additional cellular infiltration that is characteristic of this inflammatory process. Contrast enhancement in MS serves as a convenient marker for the events associated with macroscopic inflammation in MS [17–19], appearing at the time inflammation can be easily observed under the microscope, and lasting for the same time course, about 4 to 8 weeks in most cases (range <1–16 weeks) [Fig. 1] [20,21]. There is strong evidence, however, that weeks to months before lesions become evident on contrast-enhanced MR imaging, changes occur in the corresponding NAWM that can be detected by the quantitative MR imaging methodologies [22–26] including measures of perfusion [26]. Unfortunately, these measures to detect the earliest stages of MS lesions are not practical for evaluation of

individual patients at this time and they remain research tools.

The enhancement pattern (size, shape, solid versus ring) may be strikingly variable within and more so between patients, which is highly suggestive of a heterogeneous pathology, possibly related to the host response and severity [Fig. 2] [27–29]. Ring enhancement, for example, may suggest a more severe pathology [29]. Enhancement seen only after high (triple dose) MR imaging contrast infusion tends to be smaller and may indicate less destruction than that detected by single (standard) dose MR imaging contrast [30,31]. The correlation between pattern of enhancement, the underlying pathology, and clinical course in individual patients may not be straightforward, however, and is not well understood at this time.

Enhancement, which is associated with early lesions and inflammation in MS, is now also known to be associated with axonal injury. Biopsy and autopsy series show that acute, inflammatory MS lesions are accompanied by an impressive degree of axonal injury that includes axonal transection, in addition to the classic findings of demyelination [32]. Axonal injury, which is mostly irreversible,

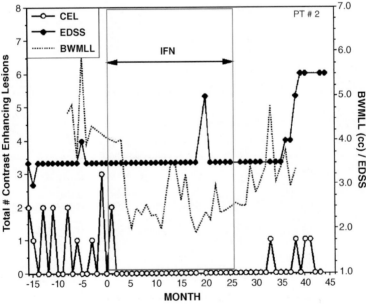

Fig. 3. High-frequency monthly MR imaging. The response to therapy may be followed by MR imaging because the MR imaging, even at yearly intervals, may suggest activity trends. In this idealized monthly MR imaging follow-up, responsiveness to initiation of therapy with interferon-β is apparent, as is return toward baseline activity with cessation of therapy. Because monthly MR imaging is not practical in the clinic, counting new T2 lesions over a 1-year interval (not shown) provides a good estimate of intercurrent MR imaging activity, because most new lesions leave a permanent T2 residue, the footprint of prior activity. Enhancing lesions at any point in time provide a measure of inflammation around the time of MR imaging. BWMLL, brain white matter lesion load; CEL, contrast-enhancing lesion number; EDSS, expanded disability status scale; IFN, interferon. (*From* Richert ND, Zierak MC, Bash CN, et al. MRI and clinical activity in MS patients after terminating treatment with interferon beta-1b. Mult Scler 2000;6:86–90; with permission.)

is an important factor even in early MS and is thought to contribute to progression to secondary progressive stages or further disability. The MR spectroscopy literature supports early axonal degeneration in the NAWM and in focal, enhancing-inflammatory lesions based on the finding of reduced *N*-acetyl aspartate (NAA), a neuronal marker [33–35].

The number and volume of enhancing lesions within individual MS patients varies over time, as most dramatically documented in high-frequency (weekly and monthly) MR imaging series [**Fig. 3**] [6,20,21]. General activity patterns, however, can often be recognized in individuals. Some individuals on most monthly enhanced MR imaging studies show little or no enhancing lesion activity, whereas others are more likely than not to have one or more lesions on most observations. These trends are used to great advantage in MS clinical trials where pooled results for many, often hundreds of patients are analyzed. Analysis based on individual patients can be informative but must be understood in the context of expected intraindividual variation over time.

Cellular imaging

Contrast enhancement suggests inflammation, but is more accurately a measure of leakage of moderate-size molecules across the damaged tight-junctions of the CNS endothelium. Cellular imaging based on superparamagnetic iron oxide–tagged cells is a more specific probe of the migration occurring at the level of the blood-brain barrier basic to the inflammatory process. In one approach, the superparamagnetic iron oxide particles after intravenous injection concentrate within macrophages and can then be followed in vivo in research studies in humans as they pass into the CNS. The intracellular particles exert a strong influence on the local magnetic field, which is detected as signal loss on T2 and T2*-weighted pulse sequences [36,37]. The location of lesions and their time-course based on superparamagnetic iron oxide imaging does not correlate strongly with that based on conventional contrast-enhanced MR imaging, suggesting that it provides different quantitative and qualitative information. In another approach, cell-type–specific tagging has been found to be feasible in animal studies. Superparamagnetic iron oxide particles are introduced outside the body into isolated cells through transfection, and the tagged cells then injected intravenously [38]. Both these cellular imaging approaches may in the near future become practical methods to monitor individual patients, and could provide far more specific detail relevant to the inflammatory process in MS. Dissecting the inflammatory process in MS is impor-

tant, because it is becoming clear that inflammation includes destructive components (bad inflammation), which clinicians want to treat, and potentially beneficial components (good inflammation), which should be enhanced or not disturbed by treatment [39,40].

The T2 hyperintense lesion

The T2 hyperintense focal areas observed on MR imaging in MS lesions are known by neuropathology studies to be caused by a wide range of pathology, and are described as nonspecific with regard to pathology. T2 hyperintensity (T2 lesions) can be the result of water space changes that include edema (acute lesions), and other water compartment changes in chronic lesions; in acute and chronic lesions mild or severe demyelination, variable degrees of astrogliosis and matrix disruption;

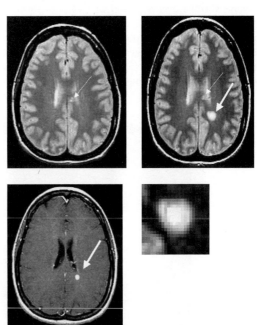

Fig. 4. Development of a T2 hyperintense lesion by serial MR imaging. Upper left: case of relapsing MS with low T2 hyperintense lesion burden including chronic lesions in the corpus callosum (*arrow*). Upper right: 1 month later, a new T2 hyperintense lesion develops in the left parietal-occipital white matter (*solid arrow*), whereas the corpus callosum lesions remain stable (*dotted arrow*). Lower left: corresponding enhancement in acute lesion (*arrow*), from blood-brain barrier breakdown and concurrent inflammation. Lower right: exploded view of the new lesion shows the complex structure, centrally hyperintense most likely from mixed pathology including demyelination, matrix including glial change, and importantly axonal degeneration. The intermediate black ring may be a zone of macrophage infiltration, and the outer ring is likely from edema.

and axonal injury or loss [**Fig. 4**] [8,17]. Complicating the interpretation of T2-weighted imaging and T2 hyperintensity, the T2 lesion areas may include zones of active remyelination [41], although remyelination is often limited and the capacity for remyelination decreases in MS with time and severity of injury.

There is increasing evidence that the underlying MS pathology is variable across patients, yet may be more homogeneous within patients (see later) [27]. Consequently pathology in an individual expressed as T2 hyperintensity may also have variable significance. This heterogeneous pathology characteristic of T2 hyperintense lesions is thought to account in part for the poor correlation between total T2 lesion volume in an individual patient's brain or spinal cord and their degree of disability [42].

After reaching a maximal lesion size over a period of about 4 to 8 weeks, the T2 hyperintensity almost always shrinks over a period of weeks to months [43], leaving a smaller residual area or T2 footprint related to the prior acute event. Although many T2 lesions do not change over years, some lesions may expand through activity along their periphery or less commonly through central activation. Re-

activation of focal lesions is thought to be an important mechanism accounting for more severe cumulative pathology, and in theory through loss of capacity for remyelination [41,44].

Over time the T2 lesion number and volume (the T2 burden of disease) increases on average in the brain or spinal cord in the absence of treatment, and most often less so when treatment is effective [**Fig. 5**]. In some individuals, the T2 burden of disease transiently decreases as lesions shrink to their footprint size and edema resolves, a finding that is not uncommon during effective treatment. With disease progression, however, lesions often become confluent because of expansion and crowding. A more minor contribution to an increasing T2 burden of disease is the result of the T2 hyperintensity that develops with secondary (fiber) degeneration that sometimes can be visualized outside focal lesions [see **Fig. 5**] [45,46]. The T2 burden of disease is an important MS trial metric, as a measure of change in total (albeit nonspecific) abnormal tissue. New or enlarging individual T2 lesions are also often measured, as an indication of new MS events within an interval between imaging studies.

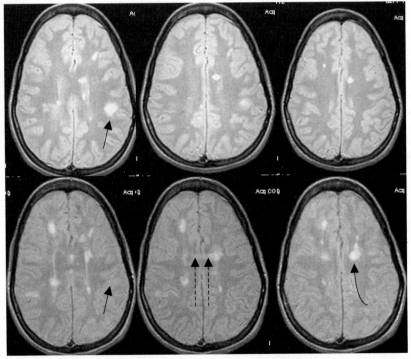

Fig. 5. Five-year follow-up after a clinically isolated syndrome shows the natural history of MS from the early stages. Proton density weighted images at three levels show accumulation of multiple new T2 hyperintense lesions and increase in T2 burden of disease. One large left frontal lesion (*arrow*) observed at baseline has shrunk leaving only a tiny T2 footprint. Note the transcallosal band (*dashed arrows*), an indication of secondary, possibly wallerian degeneration extending through the corpus callosum originating in the left frontal periventricular T2 lesion (*curved arrow*).

Chronic T1 hypointense lesions (T1 black holes)

T1-weighted imaging separates chronic MS lesions into two groups [Fig. 6]. One group of lesions, evident on T2-weighted imaging, is isointense to normal white matter on T1-weighted imaging. A smaller fraction of T2 lesions (5%–20%) are hypointense to normal white matter on T1-weighted imaging [47,48]. The chronic T1 hypointense lesion fraction (the classic T1 black hole) is important because it represents white matter that has suffered relatively more severe injury. These T1 black holes are characterized by greater reduc-

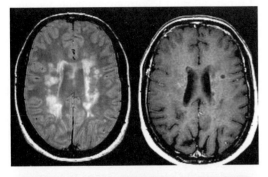

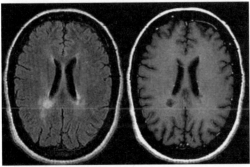

Fig. 6. Nonspecific T2 hyperintense lesions, based on comparison with postcontrast T1-weighted images that show T1 black holes. Top left shows a patient with extensive T2 hyperintense lesions, a small fraction of which (10%–20%) are T1 hypointense and nonenhancing (*right*), and considered to be classic T1 black holes. T1 black holes under the microscope characteristically are focal areas of more severe injury with loss of axons, demyelination, and matrix disruption, and show low NAA content. Bottom left shows in another patient a fast-FLAIR image with a higher ratio of T1 black hole to T2 lesion area (about 60%). The correlation between T1 black hole volume and disability tends to be slightly stronger as shown by population studies than the correlation between T2 lesion volume and disability, but in individuals T1 black hole volume is still only weakly correlated with disability. The importance of T1 black holes is that they reflect focal areas of more severe injury, and some patients may be more prone to this type of injury for reasons that are not understood.

tion in axonal density and matrix disruption as compared with T2 lesions that are not chronically T1 hypointense. These T1 black holes have relatively reduced magnetization transfer ratios (MTR), elevated diffusion coefficient, and reduced NAA, also indicative of more severe focal injury [47].

In evaluating an image, it is important to distinguish acute T1 hypointense areas, which are T1 hypointense on the basis of edema, and may show considerable or complete recovery, from chronic T1 hypointense lesions, which are the classic T1 black holes. Because serial studies are not always available to assess the chronicity of a T1 hypointense lesion, chronicity is assumed based on T1 hypointensity after contrast enhancement. High-dose corticosteroids can confound this interpretation by rapidly suppressing enhancement. In reality, acute T1 hypointense (edematous) lesions often evolve slowly over many months to their final T1 isointense or hypointense state, the latter occurring about one third of the time. Transition of an acute MS lesion to normal signal intensity on T1-weighted imaging reflects recovery from the edematous stage, and potentially partial remyelination [41]. Unfortunately, there is no specific remyelination MR imaging measure [41,44], although MTR recovery may have some potential in this regard [49].

In populations, the correlation between chronic T1 hypointense lesions and disability is thought to be stronger than the correlation between T2 lesions and disability, but the correlation is more often than not still poor. As an indication of severe injury, however, many clinicians value this parameter as a means to assess the pathologic significance of lesions (which are most often subclinical) in individuals. Chronic T1 hypointense lesion volume (T1 burden of disease) is an important MS trial measure because it is more specific than T2 burden of disease. T1 black holes are also sometimes followed in MS trials to determine if treatment has the effect of decreasing the rate of evolution of acute focal lesions to regions of severe damage [50,51].

Multiple sclerosis lesion heterogeneity by neuropathology

Recent neuropathology studies from biopsy material suggest that MS and its variants may be characterized as a heterogeneous pathology (between individuals) although relatively homogeneous within individuals [27]. The hypothesis from these studies is that the underlying pathology of MS remains a chronic T-lymphocyte–mediated inflammation, accompanied by activated macrophages and microglia and their toxic products (pattern I), but additional amplification factors generate patterns known as II, III, and IV [52]. Pattern II is based on deposition of immunoglobulins and activated complement, resembling an antibody-mediated process, and has been associated with Devic's neuromyelitis optica [53]. Pattern III is characterized by a process known as "distal dying back oligodendrogliopathy with oligodendrocyte apoptosis," and has been associated with hypoxia and perfusion abnormalities [52]. Perfusion abnormality has been recently described in MS lesions and MS NAWM [54]. There has been speculation that pattern III may also underlie Balœ's concentric sclerosis. Pattern IV, thought to be rare, is based on degeneration and oligodendrocyte death in the periplaque white matter [52]. It should be noted that this classification scheme (patterns I–IV pathology) is not free from healthy controversy [55], and is best described as a working and stimulating model for understanding MS.

Distribution of focal lesions in the brain and spinal cord

Characteristics and distribution of lesions in the brain

The characteristic distributions of focal MS lesions in the brain are well known to radiologists, and have been reviewed [8,56]. In recent years, there has been some precision added to the lesion nomenclature relevant to the new MS diagnostic criteria discussed later [57,58]. The T2 hyperintense lesions that occur throughout the CNS show a typical distribution in the periventricular (touching ventricle surface) more so than the peripheral white matter, but they occur commonly in both regions [56]. Within the white matter T2 lesions may be discrete (separate from ventricle surface), and when peripheral, many touch the gray matter (juxtacor-

tical). Lesions may straddle both gray and white matter (juxtacortical-cortical), or only rarely by MR imaging may lie entirely within the cortical gray matter (cortical). Many periventricular lesions extend at a right angle from the lateral ventricle surfaces, and have an ovoid shape reminiscent of the pathology described as Dawson's fingers, which are cellular infiltrates oriented along the periventricular veins. Infratentorial lesions are frequent in MS compared with their occurrence from small vessel disease. Deep cerebellar hemisphere, cerebellar peduncle, and brainstem surface lesions are common, the latter more typical of demyelination than infarction.

Corpus callosum lesions are frequent, and often lie within the inner or deep surfaces. Although not always seen in the earliest stages of disease, corpus callosum lesions are often early characteristic findings on MR imaging, well seen on thin section sagittal fast FLAIR sequences. These may be primary focal lesions or secondary neuronal tract lesions [46].

Optic nerve lesions are not difficult to visualize in the acute stages of optic neuritis by thin-section high-resolution fat-suppression techniques, and show strong correlations with visual function and electrophysiologic impairment [59]. In later stages, the imaging consequences of optic neuritis may only be detected by MR imaging based on atrophy or in population studies by techniques, such as magnetization transfer imaging [59]. In typical clinical optic neuritis, imaging of the optic nerve is usually not indicated, whereas a positive brain MR imaging at the time of optic neuritis may provide diagnostic criteria for possible MS [57,60] or risk for MS [61,62] or if negative suggest a low (but not zero) risk for MS [58,60]. Strong clinical MR imaging correlations are also seen for brainstem lesions causing internuclear ophthalmoplegia [63].

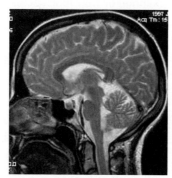 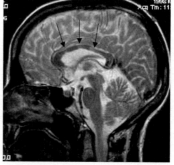

Fig. 7. Extensive corpus callosum atrophy over a 1-year interval. Note that volume loss is most extensive in the region of each T2 hyperintensity (*arrows*), but also is generalized. Atrophy in MS in the brain is likely multifactorial but based on autopsy series and MR spectroscopy thought to be principally from axonal loss. Loss of myelin and changes in the glia and water spaces likely also affect tissue volume.

Brain atrophy, often apparent on inspection in midrelapsing stages of MS, is not a rare or a late event in MS, and may progress at a surprisingly rapid pace in some individuals. In population studies, atrophy can be measured over 1-year intervals [9–11]. CNS atrophy detected by MR imaging in MS can be focal or regional affecting the central white matter and resulting in ventricular expansion or corpus callosum atrophy [**Fig. 7**], may affect the cerebellum or result in sulcal widening, and can cause global brain volume loss [64]. Atrophy is considered an important measure in MS because it likely reflects in most cases irreversible injury, much of which is from axonal loss, but additionally with contributions from myelin loss and other structural changes (those from astrogliosis) also contributory. Under relatively extreme conditions (dehydration, corticosteroid usage, malnutrition), visible atrophy may reflect reversible factors.

Characteristics and distribution of lesions in the spinal cord

Most patients with early MS have lesions within the spinal cord [65,66]. In one study of 115 patients who had optic neuritis, only 12% had an abnormal spinal cord MR imaging when the brain MR imaging was normal. However, an abnormal spinal cord was found in 45% of patients with nine or more brain lesions, the latter group known to be at higher risk for a second attack and a diagnosis of clinical MS [67].

Because spinal cord T2 hyperintense lesions are relatively rare incidental findings, and not typically observed with normal aging, in contrast to the frequent nonspecific brain T2 hyperintensities, their observation and typical features can be helpful in increasing confidence in a diagnosis of MS [**Fig. 8**] [66]. On sagittal imaging, most T2 hyperintense MS lesions in the spinal cord are vertically oriented and less than 10 to 15 mm in height or less than two vertebral segments [66]. On axial T2-weighted images, lesion distribution across the spinal cord is typically (but not always) asymmetric, corresponding to the frequent asymmetric clinical presentation of partial transverse myelitis. Acute spinal cord lesions might be expected to enhance; however, enhancement is frequently not seen probably related to technical issues and structural considerations. Chronic T1 black holes are rare in the spinal cord in MS. A diffusely swollen, T1 hypointense spinal cord is more characteristic of Devic's neuromyelitis optica [53,68] or viral or idiopathic myelitis rather than MS [**Fig. 9**]. Acute disseminated encephalomyelitis may also show an impressively swollen spinal cord. A focally swollen spinal cord, for example over one segment, although rare, occurs with sufficient frequency in

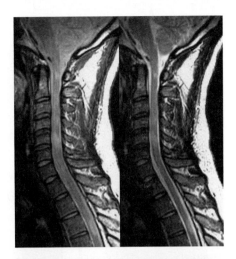

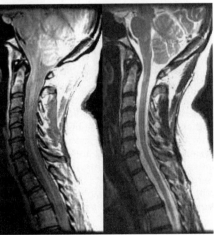

Fig. 8. MS in the spinal cord. Two patients with primary progressive MS. Top left (proton density) and top right (heavily T2-weighted) images show intrinsic multifocal T2 hyperintensities, which are vertically oriented and less than 2 vertebral segments in length. Axial sections in MS most often show an asymmetric distribution across the cord. These findings are typical for both relapsing and progressive forms of MS. Bottom left (proton density) and right (heavily T2-weighted) images show that the proton density series is frequently more sensitive to spinal cord pathology, showing both multifocal lesions and a diffuse cord hyperintensity (higher signal than cerebrospinal fluid). These findings are typical for relapsing and progressive forms of MS, but diffuse hyperintensity has been described as more common in primary progressive MS.

MS at clinical onset that this finding should not discourage consideration of MS in the differential. Brain MR imaging is often diagnostic in that setting. Later secondary changes in the spinal cord from MS include focal and diffuse volume loss [9,11,65,69,70], the atrophy related to demyelination and more so axonal loss in focal lesions, and

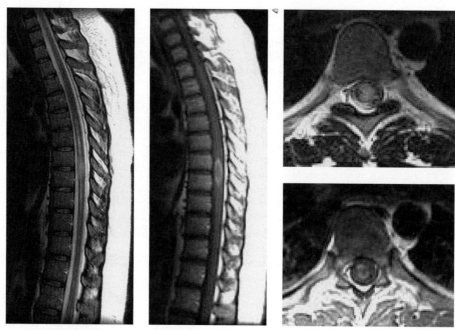

Fig. 9. Devic's neuromyelitis optica (DNO). This patient presented with bilateral visual symptoms related to demyelinating lesion of optic chiasm, and only later development of spinal symptoms. Brain white matter was otherwise normal. Sagittal images of the spinal cord show extensive thoracic cord T2 hyperintense lesion more than 2 segments in height with a cavitary enhancing pattern. The axial images show involvement of much of the cross-section of the cord. The length, ring enhancement, T1 hypointense core, and full-thickness involvement on axial images are all uncharacteristic for MS. Recent studies suggest that most but not all DNO patients are positive for a serum neuromyelitis optica (NMO)-IgG marker, whereas most MS patients are negative. The serum autoantibody data and MR imaging findings, such as normal initial brain MR imaging, support the concept that NMO is not simply an unusual manifestation of MS, and these findings expedite early aggressive therapy for DNO, which has a relatively poor prognosis.

secondary to wallerian degeneration from distant lesions [71–73].

The normal-appearing white and gray matter

From the pathology literature and now from the MR imaging literature much of the injury in MS seems to reside in the NAWM [12,49,74] and the NAGM, collectively referred to as the normal-appearing brain tissue. In the NAWM microglial inflammatory pathology may exceed that of lymphocytic inflammatory pathology, the latter so characteristic of focal lesions [12]. Axonal loss and loss or disruption of myelin may also occur in the normal-appearing brain tissue [71–73,75–77]. The abnormalities of normal-appearing brain tissue, which are difficult to detect in the earliest stages of disease, seem to increase in magnitude as disease advances, and may vary in the different MS phenotypes [12,78].

The advanced quantitative MR imaging techniques are required to detect abnormalities of the normal-appearing brain tissue in vivo. Magnetization transfer imaging is sensitive to disruption of

the macromolecular environment of membrane, cells, and tissue, and has been especially valuable in characterizing the pathology in the NAWM and NAGM in MS [78]. Loss of structure, such as when myelin fragments or is destroyed, influences the structure and concentration of macromolecules and results in a reduction in the transfer of magnetization from these to the free water fractions. These changes are readily measured by MR imaging as a decrease in the MTR. MTR changes are thought principally to reflect changes in myelin, but in the complex environment of CNS tissue, the MTR change must also reflect other factors, such as those from axonal injury and inflammation and less so edema. Typically in MS studies the average MTRs from NAWM or NAGM from groups of MS patients are evaluated using histogram analyses, based on mean MTR or other parameters, such as histogram peak height or peak location [79].

Several water diffusion-based measures also are sensitive to abnormality in the NAWM in MS [80,81]. Increased diffusivity is a relatively nonspecific finding, and is seen in focal MS lesions and normal-appearing brain tissue, in contrast to the reduced diffusivity (restricted diffusion) character-

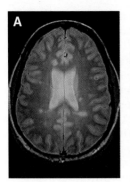 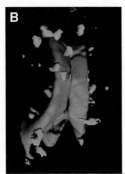 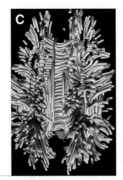 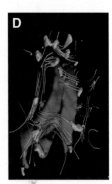

Fig. 10. Diffusion tensor imaging at 3T as basis for diffusion tractography in early relapsing MS. (*A*) The T2-weighted image reveals small lesion volume. (*B*) Computerized segmentation into lesion (*green*), ventricle (*blue*). (*C*) Stream tube tractography. The tubular structures are representations of neuronal fiber tracts with common properties that have reached a predetermined diffusion anisotropy threshold. (*D*) Final image shows only those fibers that intersect MS lesions. Note that this method allows determination as to how each lesion affects different fiber pathways, many coursing through the corpus callosum, others intersecting fibers running anteroposterior. Work based on collaboration between University of Colorado Brain Imaging Research Laboratory (J. Simon, D. Miller, M. Brown); Department of Neurology (J. Bennett and J. Corboy); and the Computer Science Department, Brown University (Song Zhang and David Laidlaw).

istic of cerebral infarction. Although cellular infiltrates characteristic of acute inflammation may counter increases in the apparent diffusion coefficient in MS lesions [80], the diffusion changes are not sufficiently specific to substitute for contrast-enhanced MR imaging. By measuring the directional components of water diffusion, the fractional anisotropy (the relative anisotropic compared with isotropic contribution) or alternatively the parallel (to fiber) versus perpendicular (to fiber) components of diffusion can be determined. Loss or decrease in anisotropy is a more specific finding than diffusivity changes in MS. Decreased anisotropy is characteristic of focal white matter MS lesions and diffuse abnormality of the NAWM. Although initially myelin was thought to be the basis for the strong diffusion anisotropy character-

istic of white matter, it now seems that organized cellular orientation rather than myelin alone may account for much of the anisotropy measured in vivo [82]. Diffusion anisotropy is the basis for diffusion tractography, which can be used as a research measure to identify the relationship between focal MS lesions and the neuronal tracts they intersect [Fig. 10].

The fundamental T1 (longitudinal) and T2 (transverse) relaxation rate measures are also sensitive to the underlying pathology in the NAWM. With specialized multiecho pulse sequences, it can be seen that T2 relaxation is multiexponential. The short T2 relaxation time fraction provides a measure that most likely is related to myelin content (myelin water fraction); a mid T2 relaxation time fraction is associated with other (interstitial) water;

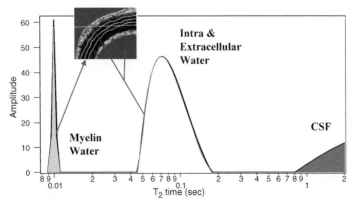

Fig. 11. Myelin water fraction. Myelin water fraction can be determined using a specialized multiecho fast spin echo pulse sequence. Analysis of the MR imaging data shows three water fractions in brain: (1) the short T2 time fraction representing myelin water, (2) the intermediate fraction intracellular and extracellular water, and (3) the long T2 time fraction cerebrospinal fluid water. The myelin water fraction is decreased in the NAWM in MS and in focal lesions (not shown). (Courtesy of C. Laule, PhD, University of British Columbia, Vancouver, Canada.)

free water produces a long T2 relaxation time fraction [**Fig. 11**] [83,84]. A current practical limitation of this method is the long scan time for full brain coverage.

By MR spectroscopy, abnormally low NAA levels can be detected in the NAWM in both relapsing and progressive MS, generally more so in the latter [12,34,35,85,86]. A recent study suggests that in the early stages of disease increased *myo*-inositol may be found in the NAWM, more so than decreased NAA [87]. As in relapsing MS, *myo*-inositol and creatine are potentially relevant to the pathology from abnormal glial cells, the latter possibly accounting for their increased concentration in the NAWM [12,87,88].

Perfusion abnormalities in the NAWM may be relevant to MS clinical or pathologic subtypes [27,52]. Decreased perfusion reflecting microvascular change or injury has been detected in the NAWM in MS [54]. Increased perfusion precedes the development of enhancing lesions in the NAWM [26]. Other quantitative MR imaging measures (MTR, relaxation measures) are also sensitive to this pre-enhancing lesion pathology in the NAWM [22–26].

The quantitative MR imaging technologies are not commonly used and are not generally helpful in evaluating individual MS patients. Rarely, MR spectroscopy may be helpful in establishing tumefactive MS versus neoplasm, but metabolite ratios or magnitude often overlap. There are reports of normal NAWM in acute disseminated encephalomyelitis and early Devic's neuromyelitis [89,90], in contrast to abnormal NAWM in MS, but these observations are based on significant differences in pooled results from multiple patients and may not be applicable to individual patients.

MR imaging is insensitive to the focal gray matter pathology of MS that is well known from the pathology literature [91], although with effort focal lesions can be seen [**Fig. 12**]. Poor tissue contrast is thought to be the basis for this MR imaging insensitivity. Focal cortical lesions often involve the subcortical white matter with only about 15% to 25% exclusively cortical [92,93], including lesions extending from the pial surface into the cortex that are never seen by conventional MR imaging [94,95]. The pathology of gray matter MS lesions is different from that seen in white matter, with gray matter MS lesions being less inflammatory with fewer lymphocytes, with fewer activated microglia, and perivascular cuffs [94,95]. These gray matter lesions, however, may contain significant destructive pathology with transected neurites (axons and dendrites) and loss of neurons from apoptosis [93]. Diffuse gray matter abnormality may also be present, because the quantitative MR imaging techniques find abnormal (but normal appearing) cortical gray matter in all MS phenotypes and stages of disease [12].

Deep gray matter involvement may also occur in MS, but disproportionate focal or diffuse T2 hyperintense or enhancing lesions in the deep gray matter suggests alternative diagnoses. Diffuse deep gray matter involvement in MS may be apparent based on volume loss [96], or by low signal on T2- or T2*-weighted imaging, which reflects increased hemosiderin or ferritin iron [97]. MS population studies suggest modest clinical correlations with this so-called "black T2" in the deep gray matter, which has potential as a neurodegeneration marker [98].

Axonal injury and neuronal tract degeneration

MS is the classic example of a primary demyelinating disorder, but demyelination alone does not account for the persistent functional disturbances that characterize the disease as it progresses. Experi-

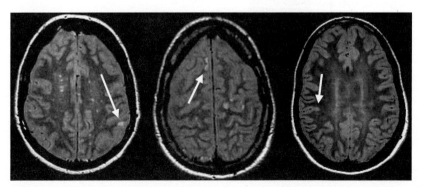

Fig. 12. Gray matter (cortical) MS. Pure cortical gray matter lesions are relatively rare by conventional MR imaging, but not uncommon by histopathology. Left panel (*arrow*) shows a focal T2 lesion centered on gray matter. Middle panel (*arrow*) shows a lesion that straddles gray and white matter (juxtacortical-cortical). Right panel (*arrow*) shows a juxtacortical (touching cortex) white matter lesion, a common finding in MS.

mental studies have shown that after myelin is damaged, nerve conduction properties, initially abnormal, can recover in part related to redistribution of sodium channels [99]. A missing link in the understanding of irreversible injury could be filled by axonal injury. Axonal injury in MS, known from the work of Charcot in the mid nineteenth century but subsequently associated only with late disease, was recently rediscovered as an important early pathology of considerable importance in MS through studies that showed convincingly that axons were in fact injured in early inflammatory MS lesions. Axonal injury was documented based on two observations: inflammatory MS lesions were associated with increases in amyloid precursor protein as a result of reduction in axonal transport from the axonal injury [100], and direct three-dimensional visualization of axonal injury in inflammatory lesions by confocal microscopy of immunostained material, which showed loss of normal neurofilament and transected axons [75]. This and subsequent work indicated that axonal injury occurred in early lesions and potentially in early MS, and it was understood immediately that axonal injury was potentially an important factor in irreversible injury, disability, and the progressive stages of disease [101].

Researchers also quickly understood the potential for such injuries to contribute to the diffuse pathology in MS through retrograde and antegrade neuronal degeneration, originating in the focal lesions but extending outside the lesion. In vivo, acute enhancing (inflammatory) MS lesions can be the source of signal and anatomic changes suggestive of secondary wallerian (fiber) degeneration [45,46]. One informative case report linked an inflammatory MS lesion in the brainstem to distant spinal cord axonal degeneration [73]. Further support for neuronal tract degeneration in MS comes from in vivo studies showing reduced NAA [102] and increased diffusivity potentially related to connected lesions [103], studies showing reduced fractional anisotropy remote from focal lesions [80], and reduced NAA in visual pathways [104].

Axonal loss can be profound in later stages of disease. In one study, there was a 53% reduction in axonal number in the NAWM of corpus callosum, which was proportionate to the reduction in cross-sectional area [105,106]. Reductions in nerve fiber density are also seen in spinal cord, including in otherwise normal-appearing tissue [72], and likely related to permanent disability [107]. Studies of fiber degeneration and connections between lesions and fiber pathways are becoming feasible in the clinical imaging environment through diffusion tensor MR imaging [see Fig. 10].

Functional MR imaging, plasticity, and adaptive mechanisms

Functional MR imaging methodologies are increasingly used to detect and explain sensorimotor and cognitive disturbances in MS. The most consistent finding by functional MR imaging studies in populations of patients with MS is impairment in sensorimotor activation indicated by abnormally increased contralateral blood oxygenation level dependent activation over larger than normal cortical regions, and increased ipsilateral supplementary motor activation [108]. Several studies suggest that sensorimotor functional MR imaging is sensitive even in the early stages of disease [109]. In secondary progressive MS [110] strong correlations have been noted between cortical activation and diffuse injury in the NAWM and NAGM. Disturbances in cognitive function including information processing can also be evaluated by functional MR imaging [111–113]. Functional disturbances detected through functional MR imaging have been the basis for hypotheses suggesting that compensatory mechanisms develop in early MS, which initially may mask injury and delay the appearance of dysfunction. Functional disturbance may only become apparent after exhaustion of these adaptive mechanisms [114–116]. Although abnormal functional MR imaging patterns may be observed in individual MS patients, their interpretation may not be straightforward, and this technique is not generally used in the clinic.

Disease course by MR imaging

At the time of the first clinical event, the CIS, many patients have multiple, previously unsuspected and widely distributed lesions in the brain or spinal cord, primarily in clinically silent areas of the white matter. These individuals are at high risk for a subsequent clinical attack or show new MR imaging evidence for ongoing demyelination, which has been recently recognized as indicative of a diagnosis of MS (see later). Alternatively, at the time of a CIS, a negative brain (and spinal cord) MR imaging suggests a low, but not zero probability of second clinical attack or MR imaging disease activity. Most of these individuals with negative MR imaging remain categorized as CIS even after prolonged clinical follow-up [117]. Although there can be striking interindividual variability, most individuals with a CIS and a positive MR imaging have a small number (2 or 3–20) and volume (a few milliliters) of focal MS lesions [118] compared with the later relapsing (typically 5–15 mL) and secondary progressive stages of disease (typically 5–25 mL) [56].

In the earliest stages of disease, focal lesions are readily counted, confluent lesions are small or relatively rare, T1 black hole volume is low, and most cases show no signs of atrophy by visual criteria. Enhancing lesions in the brain are observed in about 30% to 60% of these patients [6]. The literature is not consistent regarding the degree of abnormality of the NAWM in early MS defined at the time of a CIS, some studies suggesting abnormality, others not, which may reflect patient selection factors, but also suggests that much of the NAWM may be normal or only minimally abnormal early on.

With clinical disease progression or greater disease duration, as patients progress through relapsing and secondary progressive stages of disease, the focal T1 and T2 lesion volume increases, lesions show an increasing tendency to become confluent, and atrophy may become apparent as thinning of the corpus callosum and enlarged third and lateral ventricles [11]. Some but not all studies suggest an increase in the relative T1 black hole lesion volume with an increase in the T1/T2 lesion volume ratio. The likelihood of finding enhancing lesions on one examination in relapsing MS is similar to earlier stages of disease, ranging from about 50% to 65% in the larger studies [6]. Enhancing lesion number and volume decrease in secondary progressive MS, in parallel to the well-known decrease in clinical relapses, with enhancing lesions occurring in about 36% to 48% of patients [6].

Primary progressive multiple sclerosis

Primary progressive MS has several distinct clinical, neuropathologic, and immunologic features compared with relapsing and secondary progressive MS [119–122], but by MR imaging there is overlap with relapsing and secondary progressive MS such that by imaging alone these MS phenotypes are indistinguishable [123]. Patients classified as primary progressive on average have a decreased number and volume of enhancing lesions, which is believed to be related to the less intense inflammation observed by histopathology [120,123,124]. Spinal cord pathology has been hypothesized to be an important factor in disease progression in primary progressive MS, yet whereas patients may have severe and progressive disability localized to the spinal cord, the number or volume of T2 hyperintense spinal cord lesions does not always account for this difference in all cases [see **Fig. 8**]. Although not a distinguishing feature, there have been observations of increase in total T2 lesion volume based on expansion of pre-existing lesions more so than by additional lesions in primary progressive MS, and more diffuse rather than focal abnormality of

the spinal cord in some patients [see **Fig. 8**] [65]. Although total T2 burden of disease may be lower on average in primary progressive MS, T2 lesion measures remain the principle clinical trial measures in primary progressive MS, with atrophy measures taking on new importance [125,126].

The clinical significance of the MR imaging pathology

Acute relapse in MS is essentially an inflammatory event [127]. MS relapse early in the disease may often show good or full clinical recovery, but many relapses leave some residual deficit [128]. Inflammatory, enhancing MS lesions, when they occur in functionally eloquent regions of the CNS, result in imaging findings, symptoms, and electrophysiologic disturbances with a similar time course [129]. Most often, however, the correlation between new enhancing lesions and new clinical activity is poor, with about 5 to 10 MR imaging events on average occurring for every clinical event [130], and cases with 50 to 100 MR imaging events have been observed in the absence of any new clinical signs or symptoms [131].

Over short intervals (years), most studies find no or minimal relationships between enhancing lesions and disability. The relationship between enhancing lesions and significant injury, evidenced by atrophy, has been noted in some but not other series, but this too remains only weak at best [6,9]. One factor potentially accounting for this poor clinical (and pathology) relationship despite pathophysiologic connections is the location of lesions; for example, lesions occurring in relatively silent white matter may have only late effects when critical levels of injury (eg, fiber loss) occur, which may take years. Another factor is that much of the enhancing lesion burden may be missed with conventional imaging sensitive to only the macroscopic lesions. Also, injury associated with enhancement is likely heterogeneous and of variable severity, and measures do not account for this. Nevertheless, enhancing lesions do provide a measure of disease, with pathologic consequences, that is missed based on clinical evaluation alone.

The correlation between T2 lesion burden of disease and physical disability in population studies is significant, but very poor, and in individuals typically the relationship between lesion burden and disability can be strikingly poor. The MR imaging disability discrepancy is most likely multifactorial, related to the lack of pathologic specificity of the T2 lesion, imperfections of the disability scoring systems, and limited long-term observations. The latter is supported because the 14-year follow-up study of patients presenting initially with a CIS found a modest correlation between increasing T2 lesion load and disability [117]. The relationship between T2 burden of disease and neuropsychologic impairment is also modest at best, and in many studies poor [132].

Several studies suggest a stronger correlation between injury, indicated through the advanced quantitative MR imaging measures, and disability and cognitive dysfunction, compared with the T2 burden of disease measures. But these advanced measures in larger studies still provide only a modest at best correlation [12]. The strongest correlations between MR imaging measures and disability may be those provided by atrophy measures [132–134]. Although the limited MR imaging functional correlations are discouraging, the poor correlations may only realistically reflect the complex relationships between the pathology; its location and heterogeneity (severity); the long-term consequences that are not evaluated; and the limited measures of dysfunction (typically physical rather than cognitive or functional) that are usually used.

MR imaging in the diagnosis of multiple sclerosis

The classic diagnosis of relapsing MS until recently was based on demyelinating events occurring with dissemination in space (multiple anatomic regions) and dissemination in time based on clinical signs or symptoms. In 2001, however, new so-called "International Panel Criteria," also known as the "McDonald Criteria," were published for the diagnosis of MS [57]. The International Panel Criteria are applicable in individual patients; are well known to the neurologic community; are well (although not universally) accepted; and most important have several advantages in the early diagnosis of MS, including increased specificity and earlier diagnosis.

The International Panel Criteria are summarized in Box 1. After a clinically isolated syndrome, they are based on characteristic lesions and lesion distribution, and allow new MR imaging lesions in lieu of waiting for a second clinical attack. The latter is a key advance because substitution of an MR imaging–documented pathologic event has the potential to expedite diagnosis by months, years, or a lifetime, in contrast to requiring a second clinical event [Fig. 13]. Several studies have addressed the validation of these criteria [60]. They establish that earlier diagnosis is a frequent benefit of use of the International Panel Criteria, which allows earlier treatment in many instances, and improved counseling and support. In addition, the relatively specific dissemination in space criteria based on MR imaging can be useful in minimizing

---

Box 1: Summary of International Panel Criteria for diagnosis of multiple sclerosis after a clinically-isolated syndrome

MR imaging criteria for dissemination in space (3 of 4 of the following)[a]
1. 1 gadolinium-enhancing lesion or 9 T2-hypertense lesions if there is no gadolinium-enhancing lesion
2. ≥1 infratentorial lesion
3. ≥1 juxtacortical lesion
4. ≥3 periventricular lesions

MR imaging criteria for dissemination in time (DIT)
1. If a first scan occurs ≥3 months after the onset of the clinical event, the presence of a gadolinium-enhancing lesion is sufficient to demonstrate DIT, provided that it is not at the site implicated in the original clinical event. If there is no enhancing lesion at this time, a follow-up scan is required. The timing of this follow-up scan is not crucial, but 3 months is recommended. A new T2- or gadolinium-enhancing lesion at this time then fulfills the criterion for DIT.
2. If the first scan is performed <3 months after the onset of the clinical event, a second scan ≥3 months after the clinical event showing a new gadolinium-enhancing lesion provides sufficient evidence for DIT; however, if no enchancing lesion is seen at this second scan, a further scan not <3 months after the first scan that shows a new T2 or enhancing lesion suffices.

[a] One spinal cord lesion can be substituted for one brain lesion.
Data from McDonald WI, Compston A, Edan G, et al. Recommended diagnostic criteria for multiple sclerosis: guidelines from International Panel on the diagnosis of multiple sclerosis. Ann Neurol 2001;50(1):121–7.

---

false-positive diagnoses related to incidental nonspecific T2 hyperintensities.

The basis for the new criteria were studies that showed that at the time of a CIS, a negative MR imaging study suggests a low (up to 20%), but not zero probability of a future second attack and a formal diagnosis of MS, whereas a positive MR imaging was associated with high probability of a second attack and a formal diagnosis of MS, ranging from about 50% to 90% of cases [57]. Operational refinements in the criteria evolved with observations suggesting that the number and volume of T2 lesions at the time of a CIS, the presence of enhancing lesions, and the characteristics of the lesions (location) also increased the specificity of the various criteria [57,58,60], increased accuracy, and limited false-positive diag-

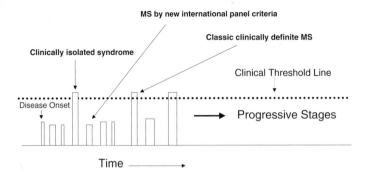

Fig. 13. Overview of relapsing-remitting MS. Vertical open bars represent MR imaging or pathologic events. Dotted line is a theoretical threshold above which lesions are clinically evident to the patient or physician. Before the first clinical event (the time of the clinically isolated syndrome), there are nearly always multiple subclinical pathologic events. Prior criteria required a second clinical event to establish a diagnosis of clinically definite MS (CDMS). By the new international panel criteria, an appropriate MR imaging event may substitute for a second clinical event in establishing dissemination in time, often expediting diagnosis. Most patients have less than one relapse per year. MR imaging events occur on average 5 to 10 times as frequently. After 5 to 10 years, most patients enter a secondary progressive stage of disease, characterized by increasing disability yet fewer relapses and focal MR imaging events.

noses, however, at the expense of sensitivity. Because a positive cerebrospinal fluid also predicts second clinical attack after a CIS, in cerebrospinal fluid–positive patients the dissemination in space criteria can be relaxed to only two MR imaging lesions according to the International Panel Criteria. Lesions in the spinal cord may substitute for lesions in the brain.

An alternative approach used by many MS neurologists in North America is to initiate therapy (in patients at risk for MS) based on positive MR imaging after a CIS, with the MR imaging positive based on at least two MR imaging lesions (periventricular or ovoid and at least 3 mm diameter), or three or more lesions [61]. The likelihood of ongoing demyelination in carefully selected individuals with a classic CIS and only a few MR imaging lesions is supported by results from the placebo arm of the CHAMPS Trial [62], which found that more than 50% of the patients not meeting the formal dissemination in space criteria of the International Panel still developed a second attack or had evidence for ongoing demyelination based on new MR imaging lesions. Although relaxed criteria (fewer lesions, less formal anatomic characteristics) increase sensitivity and function well in formal trial settings, their use must be balanced against the possibility in clinical practice of increasing false-positive diagnoses in patients with nonspecific findings, including those associated with aging and small vessel disease [60,135]. Irrespective of the criteria that are used, a careful plan for MR imaging and clinical follow-up may be informative for any patient after a first attack with a positive MR imaging study, and may reduce the likelihood of delayed diagnosis or treatment in individuals with early subclinical disease, most importantly in those with aggressive disease.

Monitoring patients by MR imaging

Practice patterns for MR imaging after the diagnosis is made are varied, ranging from never acquiring an MR imaging study unless there is a clinical concern to annual MR imaging surveillance for subclinical activity, irrespective of the clinical course. In the clinic, where monthly MR imaging [see Fig. 3] is not feasible, MR imaging activity can be monitored based on counting new T2 hyperintense lesions as a measure of interval change (eg, on annual MR imaging examinations) and counting enhancing lesions at each study as a measure of inflammation around the time of the MR imaging evaluation. Because most enhancing lesions leave a T2 footprint, counting new T2 lesions provides a reasonable estimate of new lesions that could have been more accurately determined by monthly MR imaging.

Several initiatives are underway to define criteria for successful or acceptable treatment versus treatment failure, based on both clinical and MR imaging activity [136]. Standardized MR imaging (see later) improves the accuracy of these interval assessments, and can be useful in assessing if the International Panel Criteria are met for diagnosis. Complicating the MR imaging interpretation, in addition to intraindividual variation in activity over time independent of treatment, the current therapies are only partially effective. Consequently, it may be impossible to differentiate partial but good responses (decreased lesions) versus poor responses to treatment. MR imaging monitoring, however, may increase confidence in a clinical impression of stable disease or help discount borderline symptoms or signs, supporting maintenance of the current therapy. Severe MR imaging activity may support a clinical impression or uncover a need to initiate aggressive and more risky therapy with immunosuppressive agents.

It is known that interferon-β may decrease enhancing lesions within weeks of initiation of therapy. There are only limited data regarding washout of effect after cessation of therapy, but one study found washout (return to active MR imaging disease) by 6 to 10 months after treatment with interferon beta-1b once halted [137]. Glatiramer acetate also suppresses enhancing lesions, the effect increasing to maximum benefit after an interval of about 4 to 6 months [138]. In phase II trials Tysirabi reduced enhancing and new T2 lesions in weeks [139,140]. High-dose corticosteroids may decrease enhancement within hours of administration, the effect lasting for weeks to months [141].

Clinical imaging technique

CT imaging is now used only in patients who are not appropriate subjects for MR imaging, or for indications unrelated to MS. There are multiple reasonable approaches to MR imaging for MS, and as a result there is a great deal of variability within and between institutions as to how the examination is acquired. Unfortunately, this creates a situation in which comparison of current with prior MR imaging studies can be compromised. With the more specific International Panel and other criteria, standardization can be helpful and ensure stability in decision-making over time. As a result, standardized MR imaging criteria for MS have been promoted for diagnosis and follow-up [142]. Elements of the standardized MR imaging include use of internal landmarks for setting slice location and angle; pulse sequences that are sensitive to MS pathology and comparable from scan-to-scan; and uniform standards for contrast administration including dose and sufficient interval from injection to scan. Triple-dose MR imaging contrast, delayed imaging after contrast administration, and magnetization transfer pulse sequences all increase the yield of enhancing lesions [143], but these are not required for good-quality clinical evaluation, and are not incorporated in the new MS diagnostic criteria.

The advanced quantitative imaging techniques, although invaluable in population studies, are not usually informative in individual patients. There are efforts, however, to develop reproducible acquisition and postprocessing methodologies that enable characterization of disease in individuals, such as measures of global atrophy or MTR and its change over time. Atrophy measures are increasingly used in MS clinical trials as a measure of irreversible injury [9,12], and this measure shows good long-term correlation with disability [134]. The advanced quantitative methodologies for evaluating the NAWM and NAGM are also being tested in formal clinical trial settings. These require stringent technical control to be useful in assessing individuals or populations over time [144].

References

[1] Goldman MD, Cohen JA. Multiple sclerosis. In: Rakel RE, Bope ET, editors. Conn's current therapy. Philadelphia: Elsevier Saunders; 2005. p. 1057–66.

[2] Noseworthy JH, Lucchinetti C, Rodriguez M, et al. Multiple sclerosis. N Engl J Med 2000;343: 938–52.

[3] Lublin FD, Reingold SC. Defining the clinical course of multiple sclerosis: results of an international survey. National Multiple Sclerosis Society (USA) Advisory Committee on Clinical Trials of New Agents in Multiple Sclerosis. Neurology 1996;46:907–11.

[4] Pittock SJ, McClelland RL, Mayr WT, et al. Clinical implications of benign multiple sclerosis: a 20-year population-based follow-up study. Ann Neurol 2004;56:303–6.

[5] Miller DH, Khan OA, Sheremata WA, et al. A controlled trial of natalizumab for relapsing-remitting multiple sclerosis. N Engl J Med 2003; 348:15–23.

[6] Simon JH. Measures of gadolinium enhancement in multiple sclerosis. In: Cohen JA, Rudick RA, editors. Multiple sclerosis therapeutics. 2nd edition. London: Martin Dunitz; 2003. p. 97–124.

[7] Miller DH, Albert PS, Barkhof F, et al. Guidelines for the use of magnetic resonance techniques in monitoring the treatment of multiple sclerosis. US National MS Society Task Force. Ann Neurol 1996;39:6–16.

[8] Simon JH. Pathology of multiple sclerosis as revealed by in vivo magnetic-resonance-based approaches. In: Herndon RM, editor. Multiple sclerosis: immunology, pathology, and pathophysiology. Ch 15. New York: Demos Medical Publishers; 2003. p. 199–213.

[9] Simon JH. Brain and spinal cord atrophy in multiple sclerosis: role as a surrogate measure of disease progression. CNS Drugs 2001;15: 427–36.

[10] Miller DH, Barkhof F, Frank J, et al. Measurement of atrophy in multiple sclerosis: pathological basis, methodological aspects and clinical relevance. Brain 2002;125:1676–95.

[11] Simon JH. Brain and spinal cord atrophy in

multiple sclerosis. Neuroimaging Clin N Am 2000;10:753–70.

[12] Miller DH, Thompson AJ, Filippi M. Magnetic resonance studies of abnormalities in the normal appearing white matter and grey matter in multiple sclerosis. J Neurol 2003;250:1407–19.

[13] Filippi M, Dousset V, McFarland HF, et al. Role of magnetic resonance imaging in the diagnosis and monitoring of multiple sclerosis: consensus report of the White Matter Study Group. J Magn Reson Imaging 2002;15:499–504.

[14] Sage MR, Wilson AJ, Scroop R. Contrast media and the brain: the basis of CT and MR imaging enhancement. Neuroimaging Clin N Am 1998;8:695–707.

[15] Markovic-Plese S, McFarland HF. Immunopathogenesis of the multiple sclerosis lesion. Curr Neurol Neurosci Rep 2001;1:257–62.

[16] Oksenberg JR, Baranzini SE, Hauser SL. Emerging concepts of pathogenesis: relationship to therapies for multiple sclerosis. In: Cohen JA, Rudick RA, editors. Multiple sclerosis therapeutics. 2nd edition. London: Martin Dunitz; 2003. p. 289–322.

[17] Bruck W, Bitsch A, Kolenda H, et al. Inflammatory central nervous system demyelination: correlation of magnetic resonance imaging findings with lesion pathology. Ann Neurol 1997;42:783–93.

[18] Katz D, Taubenberger JK, Cannella B, et al. Correlation between magnetic resonance imaging findings and lesion development in chronic, active multiple sclerosis. Ann Neurol 1993;34:661–9.

[19] Nesbit GM, Forbes GS, Scheithauer BW, et al. Multiple sclerosis: histopathologic and/or CT correlation in 37 cases at biopsy and three cases at autopsy. Radiology 1991;180:467–74.

[20] Lai M, Hodgson T, Gawne-Cain M, et al. A preliminary study into the sensitivity of disease activity detection by serial weekly magnetic resonance imaging in multiple sclerosis. J Neurol Neurosurg Psychiatry 1996;60:339–41.

[21] Cotton F, Weiner HL, Jolesz FA, et al. MRI contrast uptake in new lesions in relapsing-remitting MS followed at weekly intervals. Neurology 2003;60:640–6.

[22] Goodkin DE, Rooney WD, Sloan R, et al. A serial study of new MS lesions and the white matter from which they arise. Neurology 1998;51:1689–97.

[23] Filippi M, Rocca MA, Martino G, et al. Magnetization transfer changes in the normal appearing white matter precede the appearance of enhancing lesions in patients with multiple sclerosis. Ann Neurol 1998;43:809–14.

[24] Pike GB, De Stefano N, Narayanan S, et al. Multiple sclerosis: magnetization transfer MR imaging of white matter before lesion appearance on T2-weighted images. Radiology 2000;215:824–30.

[25] Narayana PA, Doyle TJ, Lai D, et al. Serial proton magnetic resonance spectroscopic imaging, contrast-enhanced magnetic resonance imaging, and quantitative lesion volumetry in multiple sclerosis. Ann Neurol 1998;43:56–71.

[26] Wuerfel J, Bellmann-Strobl J, Brunecker P, et al. Changes in cerebral perfusion precede plaque formation in multiple sclerosis: a longitudinal perfusion MRI study. Brain 2004;127(Pt 1):111–9.

[27] Lucchinetti C, Bruck W, Parisi J, et al. Heterogeneity of multiple sclerosis lesions: implications for the pathogenesis of demyelination. Ann Neurol 2000;47:707–17.

[28] Wingerchuk DM, Lucchinetti CF, Noseworthy JH. Multiple sclerosis: current pathophysiological concepts. Lab Invest 2001;81:263–81.

[29] Morgen K, Jeffries NO, Stone R, et al. Ring-enhancement in multiple sclerosis: marker of disease severity. Mult Scler 2001;7:167–71.

[30] Filippi M, Rocca MA, Rizzo G, et al. Magnetization transfer ratios in multiple sclerosis lesions enhancing after different doses of gadolinium. Neurology 1998;50:1289–93.

[31] Tortorella C, Codella M, Rocca MA, et al. Disease activity in multiple sclerosis studied by weekly triple-dose magnetic resonance imaging. J Neurol 1999;246:689–92.

[32] Bjartmar C, Trapp BD. Axonal and neuronal degeneration in multiple sclerosis: mechanisms and functional consequences. Curr Opin Neurol 2001;14:271–8.

[33] Bjartmar C, Battistuta J, Terada N, et al. N-acetylaspartate is an axon-specific marker of mature white matter in vivo: a biochemical and immunohistochemical study on the rat optic nerve. Ann Neurol 2002;51:51–8.

[34] Arnold DL, De Stefano N, Narayanan S, et al. Proton MR spectroscopy in multiple sclerosis. Neuroimaging Clin N Am 2000;10:789–98.

[35] Wolinsky JS, Narayana PA. Magnetic resonance spectroscopy in multiple sclerosis: window into the diseased brain. Curr Opin Neurol 2002;15:247–51.

[36] Dousset V, Ballarino L, Delalande C, et al. Comparison of ultrasmall particles of iron oxide (USPIO)-enhanced T2-weighted, conventional T2-weighted, and gadolinium-enhanced T1-weighted MR images in rats with experimental autoimmune encephalomyelitis. AJNR Am J Neuroradiol 1999;20:223–7.

[37] Rausch M, Hiestand P, Baumann D, et al. MRI-based monitoring of inflammation and tissue damage in acute and chronic relapsing EAE. Magn Reson Med 2003;50:309–14.

[38] Anderson SA, Shukaliak-Quandt J, Jordan EK, et al. Magnetic resonance imaging of labeled T-cells in a mouse model of multiple sclerosis. Ann Neurol 2004;55:654–9.

[39] Filippi M, Falini A, Arnold DL, et al. White Matter Study GroupMagnetic resonance techniques for the in vivo assessment of multiple

sclerosis pathology: consensus report of the white matter study group. J Magn Reson Imaging 2005;21(6):669–75.

[40] Martino G, Adorini L, Rieckmann P, et al. Inflammation in multiple sclerosis: the good, the bad, and the complex. Lancet Neurol 2002;1: 499–509.

[41] Barkhof F, Bruck W, De Groot CJ, et al. Remyelinated lesions in multiple sclerosis: magnetic resonance image appearance. Arch Neurol 2003;60:1073–81.

[42] Filippi M, Paty DW, Kappos L, et al. Correlations between changes in disability and T2-weighted brain MRI activity in multiple sclerosis: a follow-up study. Neurology 1995;45: 255–60.

[43] Guttmann CR, Ahn SS, Hsu L, et al. The evolution of multiple sclerosis lesions on serial MR. AJNR Am J Neuroradiol 1995;16:1481–91.

[44] Bruck W, Kuhlmann T, Stadelmann C. Remyelination in multiple sclerosis. J Neurol Sci 2003; 206:181–5.

[45] Simon JH, Kinkel RP, Jacobs L, et al. A wallerian degeneration pattern in patients at risk for MS. Neurology 2000;54:1155–60.

[46] Simon JH, Jacobs L, Kinkel RP. Transcallosal bands: a sign of neuronal tract degeneration in early MS? Neurology 2001;57:1888–90.

[47] van Walderveen MA, Barkhof F, Pouwels PJ, et al. Neuronal damage in T1-hypointense multiple sclerosis lesions demonstrated in vivo using proton magnetic resonance spectroscopy. Ann Neurol 1999;46:79–87.

[48] Van Walderveen MA, Kamphorst W, Scheltens P, et al. Histopathologic correlate of hypointense lesions on T1-weighted spin-echo MRI in multiple sclerosis. Neurology 1998;50:1282–8.

[49] Filippi M, Rocca MA. Magnetization transfer magnetic resonance imaging in the assessment of neurological diseases. J Neuroimaging 2004; 14:303–13.

[50] Filippi M, Rovaris M, Rocca MA, et al. Glatiramer acetate reduces the proportion of new MS lesions evolving into "black holes". Neurology 2001;57:731–3.

[51] Dalton CM, Miszkiel KA, Barker GJ, et al. Effect of natalizumab on conversion of gadolinium enhancing lesions to T1 hypointense lesions in relapsing multiple sclerosis. J Neurol 2004; 251:407–13.

[52] Lassmann H. Hypoxia-like tissue injury as a component of multiple sclerosis lesions. J Neurol Sci 2003;206:187–91.

[53] Lennon VA, Wingerchuk DM, Kryzer TJ, et al. A serum autoantibody marker of neuromyelitis optica: distinction from multiple sclerosis. Lancet 2004;364:2106–12.

[54] Law M, Saindane AM, Ge Y, et al. Microvascular abnormality in relapsing-remitting multiple sclerosis: perfusion MR imaging findings in normal-appearing white matter. Radiology 2004; 231:645–52.

[55] Barnett MH, Prineas JW. Relapsing and remitting multiple sclerosis: pathology of the newly forming lesion. Ann Neurol 2004;55:458–68.

[56] Simon JH. Magnetic resonance imaging in the diagnosis of multiple sclerosis, elucidation of disease, course, and determining prognosis. In: Burks JS, Johnson KP, editors. Multiple sclerosis: diagnosis, medical management, and rehabilitation. New York: Demos Medical Publishing; 2000. p. 99–126.

[57] McDonald WI, Compston A, Edan G, et al. Recommended diagnostic criteria for multiple sclerosis: guidelines from the International Panel on the diagnosis of multiple sclerosis. Ann Neurol 2001;50:121–7.

[58] Barkhof F, Filippi M, Miller DH, et al. Comparison of MRI criteria at first presentation to predict conversion to clinically definite multiple sclerosis. Brain 1997;120(Pt 11):2059–69.

[59] Hickman SJ, Toosy AT, Jones SJ, et al. Serial magnetization transfer imaging in acute optic neuritis. Brain 2004;127(Pt 3):692–700.

[60] Miller DH, Filippi M, Fazekas F, et al. Role of magnetic resonance imaging within diagnostic criteria for multiple sclerosis. Ann Neurol 2004;56:273–8.

[61] Frohman EM, Goodin DS, Calabresi PA, et al. The utility of MRI in suspected MS: report of the Therapeutics and Technology Assessment Subcommittee of the American Academy of Neurology. Neurology 2003;61:602–11.

[62] CHAMPS Study Group. MRI predictors of early conversion to clinically definite MS in the CHAMPS placebo group. Neurology 2002; 59:998–1005.

[63] Frohman EM, Zhang H, Kramer PD, et al. MRI characteristics of the MLF in MS patients with chronic internuclear ophthalmoparesis. Neurology 2001;57(5):762–8.

[64] Pelletier D, Garrison K, Henry R. Measurement of whole-brain atrophy in multiple sclerosis. J Neuroimaging 2004;14(3 Suppl):11S–9S.

[65] Bot JC, Barkhof F, Polman CH, et al. Spinal cord abnormalities in recently diagnosed MS patients: added value of spinal MRI examination. Neurology 2004;62:226–33.

[66] Lycklama G, Thompson A, Filippi M, et al. Spinal-cord MRI in multiple sclerosis. Lancet Neurol 2003;2:555–62.

[67] Dalton CM, Brex PA, Miszkiel KA, et al. Spinal cord MRI in clinically isolated optic neuritis. J Neurol Neurosurg Psychiatry 2003;74:1577–80.

[68] Filippi M, Rocca MA, Moiola L, et al. MRI and magnetization transfer imaging changes in the brain and cervical cord of patients with Devic's neuromyelitis optica. Neurology 1999;53: 1705–10.

[69] Lin X, Tench CR, Evangelou N, et al. Measurement of spinal cord atrophy in multiple sclerosis. J Neuroimaging 2004;14(3 Suppl):20S–6S.

[70] Stevenson VL, Ingle GT, Miller DH, et al. Magnetic resonance imaging predictors of disability

in primary progressive multiple sclerosis: a 5-year study. Mult Scler 2004;10:398–401.

[71] Bergers E, Bot JC, De Groot CJ, et al. Axonal damage in the spinal cord of MS patients occurs largely independent of T2 MRI lesions. Neurology 2002;59:1766–71.

[72] Ganter P, Prince C, Esiri MM. Spinal cord axonal loss in multiple sclerosis: a post-mortem study. Neuropathol Appl Neurobiol 1999;25:459–67.

[73] Bjartmar C, Kinkel RP, Kidd G, et al. Axonal loss in normal-appearing white matter in a patient with acute MS. Neurology 2001;57:1248–52.

[74] Allen IV, McQuaid S, Mirakhur M, et al. Pathological abnormalities in the normal-appearing white matter in multiple sclerosis. Neurol Sci 2001;22:141–4.

[75] Trapp BD, Peterson J, Ransohoff RM, et al. Axonal transection in the lesions of multiple sclerosis. N Engl J Med 1998;338:278–85.

[76] Evangelou N, Konz D, Esiri MM, et al. Regional axonal loss in the corpus callosum correlates with cerebral white matter lesion volume and distribution in multiple sclerosis. Brain 2000;123(Pt 9):1845–9.

[77] Coombs BD, Best A, Brown MS, et al. Multiple sclerosis pathology in the normal and abnormal appearing white matter of the corpus callosum by diffusion tensor imaging. Mult Scler 2004;10:392–7.

[78] Filppi M, Rocca MA, Comi G. The use of quantitative magnetic-resonance-based techniques to monitor the evolution of multiple sclerosis. Lancet Neurol 2003;2:337–46.

[79] Zhou LQ, Zhu YM, Grimaud J, et al. A new method for analyzing histograms of brain magnetization transfer ratios: comparison with existing techniques. AJNR Am J Neuroradiol 2004;25:1234–41.

[80] Bammer R, Augustin M, Strasser-Fuchs S, et al. Magnetic resonance diffusion tensor imaging for characterizing diffuse and focal white matter abnormalities in multiple sclerosis. Magn Reson Med 2000;44:583–91.

[81] Werring DJ, Clark CA, Barker GJ, et al. Diffusion tensor imaging of lesions and normal-appearing white matter in multiple sclerosis. Neurology 1999;52:1626–32.

[82] Beaulieu C. The basis of anisotropic water diffusion in the nervous system: a technical review. NMR Biomed 2002;15:435–55.

[83] Laule C, Vavasour IM, Moore GR, et al. Water content and myelin water fraction in multiple sclerosis: a T2 relaxation study. J Neurol 2004;251:284–93.

[84] Whittall KP, MacKay AL, Li DK, et al. Normal-appearing white matter in multiple sclerosis has heterogeneous, diffusely prolonged T(2). Magn Reson Med 2002;47:403–8.

[85] Fu L, Matthews PM, De Stefano N, et al. Imaging axonal damage of normal appearing white matter in multiple sclerosis. Brain 1998;121:103–13.

[86] Arnold D, Matthews PM. Measures to quantify axonal damage in vivo based on magnetic resonance spectroscopy in multiple sclerosis. In: Cohen JA, Rudick RA, editors. Multiple sclerosis therapeutics. 2nd edition. London: Martin Dunitz; 2003. p. 193–205.

[87] Fernando KT, McLean MA, Chard DT, et al. Elevated white matter myo-inositol in clinically isolated syndromes suggestive of multiple sclerosis. Brain 2004;127(Pt 6):1361–9.

[88] Rooney WD, Goodkin DE, Schuff N, et al. 1H MRSI of normal appearing white matter in multiple sclerosis. Mult Scler 1997;3:231–7.

[89] Ghezzi A, Bergamaschi R, Martinelli V, et al. Clinical characteristics, course and prognosis of relapsing Devic's neuromyelitis optica. J Neurol 2004;251:47–52.

[90] Filippi M, Rocca MA, Moiola L, et al. MRI and magnetization transfer imaging changes in the brain and cervical cord of patients with Devic's neuromyelitis optica. Neurology 1999;53:1705–10.

[91] Catalaa I, Fulton JC, Zhang X, et al. MR imaging quantitation of gray matter involvement in multiple sclerosis and its correlation with disability measures and neurocognitive testing. AJNR Am J Neuroradiol 1999;20:1613–8.

[92] Kidd D, Barkhof F, McConnell R, et al. Cortical lesions in multiple sclerosis. Brain 1999;122(Pt 1):17–26.

[93] Peterson JW, Bo L, Mork S, et al. Transected neurites, apoptotic neurons, and reduced inflammation in cortical multiple sclerosis lesions. Ann Neurol 2001;50:389–400.

[94] Bo L, Vedeler CA, Nyland HI, et al. Subpial demyelination in the cerebral cortex of multiple sclerosis patients. J Neuropathol Exp Neurol 2003;62:723–32.

[95] Bo L, Vedeler CA, Nyland H, et al. Intracortical multiple sclerosis lesions are not associated with increased lymphocyte infiltration. Mult Scler 2003;9:323–31.

[96] Bermel RA, Innus MD, Tjoa CW, et al. Selective caudate atrophy in multiple sclerosis: a 3D MRI parcellation study. Neuroreport 2003;14:335–9.

[97] Schenck JF, Zimmerman EA. High-field magnetic resonance imaging of brain iron: birth of a biomarker? NMR Biomed 2004;17:433–45.

[98] Bakshi R, Benedict RH, Bermel RA, et al. T2 hypointensity in the deep gray matter of patients with multiple sclerosis: a quantitative magnetic resonance imaging study. Arch Neurol 2002;59:62–8.

[99] Waxman SG. Demyelinating diseases: new pathological insights, new therapeutic targets. N Engl J Med 1998;338:323–5.

[100] Ferguson B, Matyszak MK, Esiri MM, et al. Axonal damage in acute multiple sclerosis lesions. Brain 1997;120:393–9.

[101] Bjartmar C, Wujek JR, Trapp BD. Axonal loss

in the pathology of MS: consequences for understanding the progressive phase of the disease. J Neurol Sci 2003;206:165–71.

[102] De Stefano N, Narayanan S, Matthews PM, et al. In vivo evidence for axonal dysfunction remote from focal cerebral demyelination of the type seen in multiple sclerosis. Brain 1999; 122(Pt 10):1933–9.

[103] Werring DJ, Clark CA, Droogan AG, et al. Water diffusion is elevated in widespread regions of normal-appearing white matter in multiple sclerosis and correlates with diffusion in focal lesions. Mult Scler 2001;7:83–9.

[104] Heide AC, Kraft GH, Slimp JC, et al. Cerebral N-acetylaspartate is low in patients with multiple sclerosis and abnormal visual evoked potentials. AJNR Am J Neuroradiol 1998;19: 1047–54.

[105] Evangelou N, Esiri MM, Smith S, et al. Quantitative pathological evidence for axonal loss in normal appearing white matter in multiple sclerosis. Ann Neurol 2000;47:391–5.

[106] Evangelou N, Konz D, Esiri MM, et al. Regional axonal loss in the corpus callosum correlates with cerebral white matter lesion volume and distribution in multiple sclerosis. Brain 2000; 123(Pt 9):1845–9.

[107] Wujek JR, Bjartmar C, Richer E, et al. Axon loss in the spinal cord determines permanent neurological disability in an animal model of multiple sclerosis. J Neuropathol Exp Neurol 2002;61:23–32.

[108] Filippi M, Rocca MA, Mezzapesa DM, et al. A functional MRI study of cortical activations associated with object manipulation in patients with MS. Neuroimage 2004;21:1147–54.

[109] Filippi M, Rocca MA, Mezzapesa DM, et al. Simple and complex movement-associated functional MRI changes in patients at presentation with clinically isolated syndromes suggestive of multiple sclerosis. Hum Brain Mapp 2004;21:108–17.

[110] Rocca MA, Gavazzi C, Mezzapesa DM, et al. A functional magnetic resonance imaging study of patients with secondary progressive multiple sclerosis. Neuroimage 2003;19:1770–7.

[111] Mainero C, Caramia F, Pozzilli C, et al. fMRI evidence of brain reorganization during attention and memory tasks in multiple sclerosis. Neuroimage 2004;21:858–67.

[112] Audoin B, Ibarrola D, Ranjeva JP, et al. Compensatory cortical activation observed by fMRI during a cognitive task at the earliest stage of MS. Hum Brain Mapp 2003;20:51–8.

[113] Staffen W, Mair A, Zauner H, et al. Cognitive function and fMRI in patients with multiple sclerosis: evidence for compensatory cortical activation during an attention task. Brain 2002; 125(Pt 6):1275–82.

[114] Cifelli A, Matthews PM. Cerebral plasticity in multiple sclerosis: insights from fMRI. Mult Scler 2002;8:193–9.

[115] Filippi M, Rocca MA. Cortical reorganisation in patients with MS. J Neurol Neurosurg Psychiatry 2004;75:1087–9.

[116] Filippi M. MRI-clinical correlations in the primary progressive course of MS: new insights into the disease pathophysiology from the application of magnetization transfer, diffusion tensor, and functional MRI. J Neurol Sci 2003; 206:157–64.

[117] Brex PA, Ciccarelli O, O'Riordan JI, et al. A longitudinal study of abnormalities on MRI and disability from multiple sclerosis. N Engl J Med 2002;346:158–64.

[118] CHAMPS Study Group. Baseline MRI characteristics of patients at high risk for multiple sclerosis: results from the CHAMPS trial. Mult Scler 2002;8:332–8.

[119] Pender MP. The pathogenesis of primary progressive multiple sclerosis: antibody-mediated attack and no repair? J Clin Neurosci 2004;11: 689–92.

[120] Thompson AJ, Polman CH, Miller DH, et al. Primary progressive multiple sclerosis. Brain 1997;120:1085–96.

[121] Wolinsky JS. The diagnosis of primary progressive multiple sclerosis. J Neurol Sci 2003;206: 145–52.

[122] Bruck W, Lucchinetti C, Lassmann H. The pathology of primary progressive multiple sclerosis. Mult Scler 2002;8:93–7.

[123] Kremenchutzky M, Lee D, Rice GP, et al. Diagnostic brain MRI findings in primary progressive multiple sclerosis. Mult Scler 2000;6:81–5.

[124] Filippi M, Rovaris M, Rocca MA. Imaging primary progressive multiple sclerosis: the contribution of structural, metabolic, and functional MRI techniques. Mult Scler 2004; 10(Suppl 1):S36–44 [discussion: S44–5].

[125] Stevenson VL, Miller DH, Leary SM, et al. One year follow up study of primary and transitional progressive multiple sclerosis. J Neurol Neurosurg Psychiatry 2000;68:713–8.

[126] Leary SM, Miller DH, Stevenson VL, et al. Interferon beta-1a in primary progressive MS: an exploratory, randomized, controlled trial. Neurology 2003;60:44–51.

[127] McDonald WI. Relapse, remission, and progression in multiple sclerosis. N Engl J Med 2000; 343:1486–7.

[128] Lublin FD, Baier M, Cutter G. Effect of relapses on development of residual deficit in multiple sclerosis. Neurology 2003;61:1528–32.

[129] Youl BD, Turano G, Miller DH, et al. The pathophysiology of acute optic neuritis: an association of gadolinium leakage with clinical and electrophysiological deficits. Brain 1991; 114(Pt 6):2437–50.

[130] Barkhof F, Scheltens P, Frequin ST, et al. Relapsing-remitting multiple sclerosis: sequential enhanced MR imaging vs clinical findings in determining disease activity. AJR Am J Roentgenol 1992;159:1041–7.

[131] Jacobs LD, Beck RW, Simon JH, et al. Intramuscular interferon beta-1a therapy initiated during a first demyelinating event in multiple sclerosis. CHAMPS Study Group. N Engl J Med 2000;343:898–904.

[132] Benedict RH, Weinstock-Guttman B, Fishman I, et al. Prediction of neuropsychological impairment in multiple sclerosis: comparison of conventional magnetic resonance imaging measures of atrophy and lesion burden. Arch Neurol 2004;61:226–30.

[133] Amato MP, Bartolozzi ML, Zipoli V, et al. Neocortical volume decrease in relapsing-remitting MS patients with mild cognitive impairment. Neurology 2004;63:89–93.

[134] Fisher E, Rudick RA, Simon JH, et al. Eight-year follow-up study of brain atrophy in patients with MS. Neurology 2002;59:1412–20.

[135] Simon JH, Thompson AJ. Is multiple sclerosis still a clinical diagnosis? Neurology 2003;61:596–7.

[136] Rudick RA, Lee JC, Simon J, et al. Defining interferon beta response status in multiple sclerosis patients. Ann Neurol 2004;56:548–55.

[137] Richert ND, Zierak MC, Bash CN, et al. MRI and clinical activity in MS patients after terminating treatment with interferon beta-1b. Mult Scler 2000;6:86–90.

[138] Comi G, Filippi M, Wolinsky JS. European/Canadian multicenter, double-blind, randomized, placebo-controlled study of the effects of glatiramer acetate on magnetic resonance imaging: measured disease activity and burden in patients with relapsing multiple sclerosis. European/Canadian Glatiramer Acetate Study Group. Ann Neurol 2001;49:290–7.

[139] Miller DH, Khan OA, Sheremata WA, et al. International Natalizumab Multiple Sclerosis Trial GroupA controlled trial of natalizumab for relapsing multiple sclerosis. N Engl J Med 2003; 348:15–23.

[140] O'Connor PW, Goodman A, Willmer-Hulme AJ, et al. Randomized multicenter trial of natalizumab in acute MS relapses: clinical and MRI effects. Neurology 2004;62:2038–43.

[141] Miller DH, Thompson AJ, Morrissey SP, et al. High dose steroids in acute relapses of multiple sclerosis: MRI evidence for a possible mechanism of therapeutic effect. J Neurol Neurosurg Psychiatry 1992;55:450–3.

[142] Simon JH, Traboulsee A, et al. Standardized MRI protocol for multiple sclerosis: Consortium of MS Centers (CMSC) consensus guidelines. AJNR 2005, in press.

[143] Silver NC, Good CD, Sormani MP, et al. A modified protocol to improve the detection of enhancing brain and spinal cord lesions in multiple sclerosis. J Neurol 2001;248:215–24.

[144] Horsfield MA, Barker GJ, Barkhof F, et al. Guidelines for using quantitative magnetization transfer magnetic resonance imaging for monitoring treatment of multiple sclerosis. J Magn Reson Imaging 2003;17:389–97.

ELSEVIER
SAUNDERS

RADIOLOGIC
CLINICS
OF NORTH AMERICA

Radiol Clin N Am 44 (2006) 101–110

Imaging of Cervical Lymph Nodes in Head and Neck Cancer: The Basics

Devang M. Gor, MB, BS[a], Jill E. Langer, MD[b],
Laurie A. Loevner, MD[a],*

- Imaging characteristics: cross-sectional imaging
  - *Lymph node size and contour*
  - *Necrotic and cystic lymph nodes*
  - *Calcified nodes*
- Imaging characteristics: sonography
- What the clinician needs to know
  - *Extracapsular spread*
  - *Carotid invasion*
  - *Skull base and vertebral invasion*
- Evaluation of adenopathy with an occult primary
- Evolving techniques and contrast agents
- Tumor recurrence versus treatment changes: a job for positron emission tomography imaging?
- Summary
- References

Head and neck cancer accounts for 3% to 4% of all malignancies with approximately 65,000 new cases detected every year [1]. The male/female ratio is 2:1 with 90% of cancers representing squamous cell carcinomas. Critical to the treatment planning and prognostic assessment of these malignancies is identification of regional cervical nodal metastatic disease. Clinical palpation in malignant disease is not highly reliable with a sensitivity of 65% and an accuracy of approximately 75% [2,3]. Imaging improves accuracy to 80% to 85%, identifying pathologic cervical adenopathy in a significant number of patients with head and neck cancer who have no palpable adenopathy on physical examination [4]. For example, retropharyngeal nodes can only be identified on cross-sectional imaging. Imaging also identifies necrosis (indicative of metastatic disease) in enlarged and normal-sized nodes, although it is limited in detecting microscopic disease in normal-sized nodes. Even on initial pathologic sectioning of lymph nodes, however, metastatic disease may be missed in up to 3% of cases. This article addresses the assessment of cervical lymph nodes in head and neck cancer, emphasizing what clinicians need to know to stage and manage their patients.

The first step in assessing the neck for metastatic disease is knowledge of the nodal classification, namely the anatomic level of pathologic nodes. The American Joint Committee on Cancer Staging classifies the lymph nodes as level I through level VII [5]. Level I refers to nodes in the submandibular and submental region. Levels II, III, and IV refers to lymph nodes along the anterior cervical

[a] Division of Neuroradiology, Department of Radiology, Hospital of University of Pennsylvania, University of Pennsylvania Medical Center, Philadelphia, PA, USA
[b] Division of Ultrasonography, Department of Radiology, Hospital of University of Pennsylvania, University of Pennsylvania Medical Center, Philadelphia, PA, USA
* Corresponding author. Division of Neuroradiology, Department of Radiology, Hospital of University of Pennsylvania, University of Pennsylvania Medical Center, 3400 Spruce Street, 2nd Floor Dulles, Suite 219, Philadelphia, PA 19104.
E-mail address: laurie.loevner@uphs.upenn.edu (L.A. Loevner).

0033-8389/06/$ – see front matter © 2005 Elsevier Inc. All rights reserved.
radiologic.theclinics.com

doi:10.1016/j.rcl.2005.08.006

chain. Level V is those nodes in the posterior compartment previously referred to as the "spinal accessory chain" because they follow the spinal accessory nerve. Level VI nodes are in the visceral compartment of the neck, whereas level VIIs are in the superior mediastinum [Box 1 and **Fig. 1**].

In the assessment of regional nodal metastases in patients with head and neck cancer, the radiologist must identify if pathologic nodes are ipsilateral, contralateral, or bilateral. Pathologic lymph nodes are established either by size (enlargement) or the presence of abnormal nodal architecture. In addition, the presence of extracapsular spread of tumor, carotid encasement, and fixation of the tumor to the skull base or prevertebral space should be evaluated because these features of cancerous nodes affect prognosis and management. The presence of nodal metastases decreases the patient's morbidity and mortality by 50%; if there is bilateral lymph-

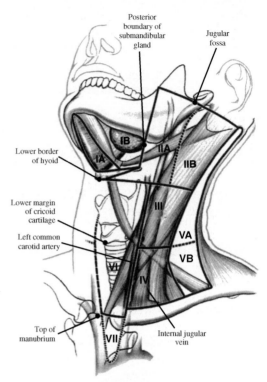

Fig. 1. Imaging classification of pathologic lymph nodes. (*From* Som PM, Curtin HD, Mancuso AA. An imaging-based classification for the cervical nodes designed as an adjunct to recent clinically based nodal classification. Arch Otolaryngol Head Neck Surg 1999; 125:388–96; with permission.)

adenopathy the patient's prognosis is reduced by another 50%; the presence of extracapsular spread reduces the patient's morbidity and mortality by another 50%; and when there is nodal fixation the prognosis is reduced further by 50%.

Imaging characteristics: cross-sectional imaging

Lymph node size and contour

The size criteria for lymph nodes that have been established are somewhat arbitrary. Using maximum longitudinal diameter, the upper limits of normal in size for lymph nodes at level I (submental and submandibular) and the jugulodigastric nodes at level II is 1.5 cm in transverse dimension. For the remaining cervical lymph node levels, 1 cm is the accepted upper limits of normal in size. There have been no large studies looking at the size criteria for retropharyngeal lymph nodes. Retropharyngeal lymph nodes are always abnormal when necrotic in the setting of cancer. In patients with pharyngeal cancer (nasopharynx, soft palate, tonsil, or base of tongue), retropharyngeal lymph nodes should be viewed with concern when they are 6 to

---

Box 1: American Joint Committee on Cancer classification of cervical lymph nodes based on level and location

Level I
  Ia: Submental
  Ib: Submandibular
Level II: Anterior cervical lymph node chain. Lymph nodes in the internal jugular chain from the skull base to the level of the hyoid bone.
  IIa: Nodes anterior, medial, or lateral to the internal jugular vein
  IIb: Nodes posterior to the internal jugular vein with a fat plane between the node and the vessel
Level III: Nodes along the internal jugular chain between the hyoid bone and the cricoid cartilage
Level IV: Nodes along the internal jugular chain between the cricoid cartilage and the clavicle
Level V: Nodes along the spinal accessory chain, posterior to the sternocleidomastoid muscle
  Va: Level V nodes from the skull base to lower border of cricoid cartilage
  Vb: Level V nodes from lower border of cricoid cartilage to the clavicle
Level VI: Nodes in the visceral compartment from the hyoid bone superiorly to the suprasternal notch inferiorly. On each side, the lateral border is formed by the medial border of the carotid sheath.
Level VII: Nodes in the superior mediastinum

Data from American Joint Committee on Cancer Staging. American Joint Committee on Cancer Staging manual. 5th edition. Philadelphia: Lippincott Raven; 1997.

8 mm in size. In the setting of papillary thyroid cancer, retropharyngeal nodes must also be carefully assessed, and if enlarged, especially with elevated thyroglobulin levels, may be aspirated with imaging guidance. It should be noted that these numbers have been somewhat arbitrarily determined, and many malignant nodes may be normal in size, whereas enlarged nodes may be benign. Lymph node shape is not specific; however, benign nodes tend to be kidney bean or flat in appearance, whereas malignant nodes tend to be rounded. Using the ratio of long axis dimension to short axis dimension has been suggested. Long axis dimension/short axis dimension >2 favors a benign node, whereas a ratio <2 is more concerning for metastatic disease [6]. The ratio depicts the fact that malignant nodes tend to be more rounded when compared with normal nodes. Size criteria alone are not reliable, with a false-positive and false-negative rate of 15% and 20%, respectively. In the assessment of nodes that are borderline by imaging criteria, knowledge of the nodal drainage patterns for a spectrum of primary cancers can be helpful in gauging ones level of suspicion.

Necrotic and cystic lymph nodes

The presence of fat within a node is usually indicative of a benign node. The hilus of lymph nodes contains fat, which may be distinguished from necrosis by its location at the periphery of the node, compared with necrosis, which occurs centrally, and its density on CT or intensity on MR imaging, which is similar to the fat in the surrounding tissues of the neck.

Identification of nodal necrosis is important and implies the presence of regional metastases until proved otherwise in patients with squamous cell carcinoma of the head and neck. Necrotic or cystic nodes are not uncommonly seen in metastatic thy-

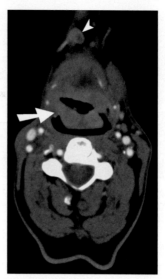

Fig. 3. Contrast-enhanced axial CT scan at the level of the base of the tongue with normal-sized but necrotic level IA lymph node (*arrowhead*) in a patient with carcinoma of the base of the tongue (*arrow*).

roid cancer, most commonly papillary carcinoma. Rarely, non-Hodgkin's lymphoma may present with necrotic lymphadenopathy (less than 4% of the time). On CT a necrotic lymph node has central low density with a thick rind of residual enhancing lymphatic tissue [Figs. 2 and 3]. On MR imaging, necrosis is identified as low signal intensity on T1-weighted images with corresponding high signal intensity on T2-weighted images with peripheral enhancement. It been suggested that CT may be slightly superior to MR imaging in the detection of nodal necrosis [7]. Recent studies, however, indicate that MR imaging has sensitivity comparable with CT, especially when using surface coils and larger matrix size, both being more sensitive when compared with ultrasonography (US). The reported accuracy, sensitivity, and specificity by CT and MR imaging range between 91% and 93%. Using US, the reported accuracy, sensitivity, and specificity are 85%, 77%, and 93%, respectively [8]. The frequency of necrosis in a metastatic lymph node increases with lymph node size, with 10% to 33% of metastatic nodes smaller than 1 cm showing necrosis and 56% to 63% of nodes larger than 1.5 cm showing necrosis [9,10].

Cystic lymphadenopathy is the term used to describe nodes completely replaced by material similar in density (CT) or intensity (MR imaging) to water (0–20 HU) with a thin or imperceptible wall [Fig. 4]. Not uncommonly, some cystic nodes have increased protein content resulting in higher attenuation on CT (HU > 20) and high signal intensity on unenhanced T1-weighted MR images. Cystic nodes are often seen in metastatic papillary thy-

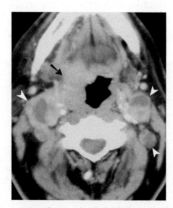

Fig. 2. Contrast-enhanced axial CT scan at the level of the base of the tongue with bilateral enlarged necrotic level II lymph nodes (*arrowheads*) in a patient with carcinoma of the base of the tongue (*arrow*).

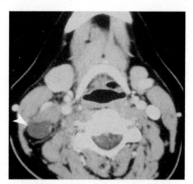

Fig. 4. Contrast-enhanced axial CT scan of the neck with a cystic level II-III lymph node (*arrowhead*) in a patient with tonsillar cancer.

roid carcinoma [**Fig. 5**]. In addition, in squamous cell cancer of the head and neck, cystic adenopathy may occur. In this setting, primary malignancies arising from the base of the tongue and tonsil should be strongly considered.

A common pitfall is to attribute a large cystic neck lesion in an adult as a branchial cleft cyst. Sometimes the distinction is difficult [**Fig. 6**]; however, detection of a cystic neck mass in an adult should prompt the radiologist to look for head and neck cancer and papillary carcinoma of the thyroid gland.

Calcified nodes

Cervical lymph node calcification is rare and is seen in about 1% of lymph nodes [11]. Presence of nodal calcification is not a reliable predictor of either benign or malignant disease; however, it does provide a limited differential diagnosis as to the possible etiology. Calcification in lymph nodes is most common in papillary thyroid cancer [**Fig. 7**]. It is occasionally seen in metastatic mu-

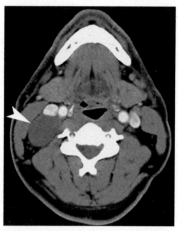

Fig. 6. Contrast-enhanced axial CT scan of the neck shows a large cystic lesion (*arrowhead*) medial to the right sternocleidomastoid muscle. Imaging features may suggest a branchial cleft cyst; however, the location is atypical for it. Pathologic examination revealed metastasis from papillary thyroid cancer.

cinous adenocarcinoma, treated lymphoma, and granulomatous disease.

Imaging characteristics: sonography

Sonography of the neck offers an inexpensive and readily available means to evaluate for cervical adenopathy; however, operator experience is important because some of the sonographic findings of malignant disease may be subtle. The examination should be performed with a high-frequency, linear transducer, preferably with Doppler capability. The central compartment of the neck and both lateral compartments should be thoroughly scanned in both transverse and longitudinal orientation. Normal nodes are commonly seen on routine examination and typically are oval or oblong in shape, with a uniform hypoechoic cortex surrounding an echogenic hilus [**Fig. 8**]. The echo-

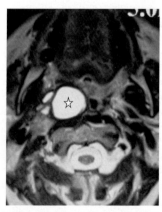

Fig. 5. Axial T2-weighted MR image at the level of nasopharynx with a large cystic right retropharyngeal lymph node (*star*) in a patient with papillary carcinoma of the thyroid gland.

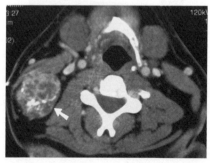

Fig. 7. Contrast-enhanced axial CT scan of the neck with necrotic calcified lymph nodes (*arrow*) in a patient with papillary carcinoma of the thyroid gland.

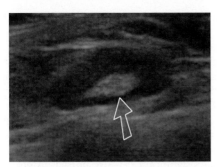

Fig. 8. Longitudinal sonogram shows an oval-shaped normal lymph node with an echogenic central hilus (*arrow*) and a uniformly hypoechoic periphery.

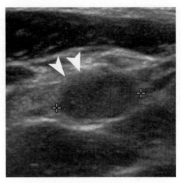

Fig. 10. Transverse sonogram showing an irregular anterior border (*arrowheads*) with possible infiltration of the adjacent connective tissue of this metastatic lymph node (*calipers*) from tall cell papillary thyroid carcinoma that proved to have extracapsular extension on surgical pathology.

genicity of the hilus had been attributed to presence of hilar fat; however, Vassallo and coworkers [12,13] determined that the appearance is caused by a large number of lymph-collecting sinuses posing numerous acoustic interfaces, reflecting the US beam. On color Doppler, normal nodes may have no detectable flow or only flow within the hilar vessels [14].

Metastatic disease may be detected by noting an increase in the short axis diameter, a change in the shape or contour, or an alteration in the consistency or internal echotexture of the affected node [15]. A rounded shape is also considered abnormal in smaller node with the exception of the submandibular and parotid nodes, which commonly appear more rounded. Focal or eccentric hypertrophy of the peripheral cortex is a useful sign to identify malignant nodes, because it usually indicates tumor infiltration and may be seen before nodal enlargement has occurred. Absence of the echogenic hilus may be useful as a sign of an abnormal lymph node, but should not be used as the sole criteria to identify abnormality because it may result from both benign and malignant causes or may be related to sonographic technique or small node size rather than a true abnormality. Increased short axis diameter and absence of cen-

tral hilar echogenicity are the criteria most predictive of metastatic involvement of lymph nodes [16,17]. Metastatic nodes are usually hypoechoic relative to muscle, with the exception of metastatic papillary carcinoma of the thyroid, which may appear hyperechoic, resembling the echogenicity of the thyroid gland [**Fig. 9**]. Identification of a hyperechoic node should prompt the operator to evaluate the thyroid gland for a possible thyroid carcinoma.

Metastatic lymph nodes tend to have a distinct margin; an indistinct margin raises the possibility of extracapsular spread of disease [**Fig. 10**]. Necrosis and cystic change are frequently seen in metastatic disease, but may also be seen in granulomatous diseases. Clinical information is vital for interpretation. A nearly entirely cystic lymph node is suspicious for metastatic papillary thyroid carcinoma [**Fig. 11**]. Microcalcification within a lymph node has been reported to occur with metastatic papillary thyroid cancer and medullary carcinoma of the thyroid gland. This is best seen with a high-frequency transducer and appears as small flecks of punctuate hyperechogenicity without acoustic

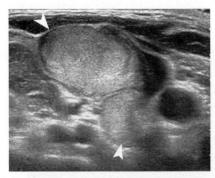

Fig. 9. Longitudinal sonogram shows two adjacent enlarged hyperechoic lymph nodes (*arrowheads*) in a patient with carcinoma of the thyroid gland.

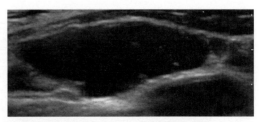

Fig. 11. This lateral cervical lymph node is nearly entirely cystic in its appearance with a few thin internal septations and a slight irregular border. A predominantly cystic lymph node in the lateral cervical chain is suspect for metastatic thyroid carcinoma.

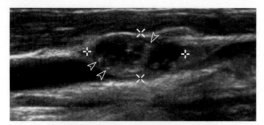

Fig. 12. Longitudinal sonogram of a lateral cervical lymph node with several punctate echogenic foci (*arrowheads*) indicating microcalcifications from metastatic papillary thyroid carcinoma. The underlying internal jugular vein is compressed but not invaded.

shadowing [**Fig. 12**]. This pattern is somewhat unique, because calcification seen in granulomatous disease or following chemotherapy or radiation tends to be larger and coarse in morphology.

Doppler US can also be used to predict further the metastatic nature of the enlarged nodes [18]. Central or hilar vascularity can be seen in normal or benign reactive nodes, whereas peripheral or combined peripheral and central hypervascularity is strongly suggestive of malignancy [**Fig. 13**]. The one exception is lymphoma, which may only have hilar flow. The use of flow patterns, such as peripheral vascularity with or without central vascularity, improves the overall accuracy of sonography to 92% in identifying metastatic nodes [19].

US-guided fine-needle aspiration can be performed to obtain cells for cytologic evaluation and confirmation of suspected metastatic disease and to obtain samples for microbiologic evaluation. US-guided fine-needle aspiration cytology has an accuracy of 95% to 97% to provide the appropriate diagnosis and is commonly used to evaluate cervical adenopathy [20,21].

What the clinician needs to know

Once the presence of regional metastases has been determined, staging is the next important step, with guidelines determined by the American Joint Committee on Cancer [Box 2]. In general, features of

lymph nodes that determine surgery include laterality, nodal size, single versus multiple nodes, and relationship to site of the primary tumor. Several additional features of nodal metastases should be communicated to the surgeon because they have a significant impact on prognosis and management. Specifically, the presence of extracapsular extension, carotid encasement or invasion, or extension or fixation to the skull base or prevertebral space may render the patient inoperable in addition to having a significant negative impact on prognosis.

Extracapsular spread

The presence of macroscopic extracapsular extension of metastatic disease increases the local recurrence rate by 3.5 times when compared with absence of nodal metastasis or metastatic adenopathy without extracapsular spread in a patient with squamous cell cancer [22]. When two or more nodes show extracapsular spread, regional recurrence rate is 58.3%, and the rate of distant metastases is 33.3% with a median survival of less than 1 year reported [23]. Lymph node size is also an indicator of extracapsular spread. Although 25% of malignant lymph nodes ≤1 cm in size may be associated with microscopic extracapsular extension, 75% of nodes >3 cm are associated with such extracapsular spread.

Extracapsular extension may be suspected when there are poorly defined nodal margins or when there is soft tissue infiltration or stranding of the muscles or fat in the neck [**Fig. 14**]. The sensitivity of CT to diagnose extracapsular spread is about 81% and the specificity about 72% [24]. The sensitivity and specificity by MR imaging ranges from 57% to 77% and 57% to 72% for extracapsular spread, respectively [25].

Carotid invasion

Preoperative identification of carotid encasement by neoplasm (primary or nodal) is important for treatment planning. In a surgical candidate, an internal carotid artery balloon occlusion test may be performed to determine if the patient is able to

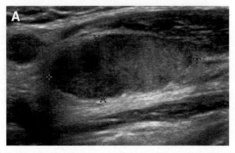

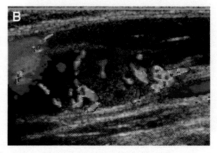

Fig. 13. (*A*) Gray scale shows an abnormal lateral cervical lymph node, which is enlarged without an echogenic central hilus. (*B*) Color Doppler examination shows multiple vessels within the node.

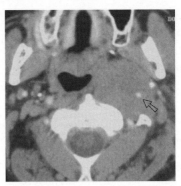

Fig. 15. Contrast-enhanced axial CT scan of the neck shows a large left retropharyngeal lymph node mass encasing the internal carotid artery (*arrow*).

tolerate sacrifice of the carotid artery if necessary in the operating room.

Carotid encasement is usually assessed by evaluating the fatty interface between the tumor and the vessel wall. The presence of tumor around the internal carotid artery by a circumference of less than 180 degrees normally indicates the absence of invasion, whereas tumor that encases the carotid artery by greater than 270 degrees is usually indicative of invasion [**Fig. 15**]. Using CT, MR imaging, or US, carotid involvement of 270 degrees or more predicted arterial wall invasion with a sensitivity of 92% to 100%, and a specificity of 88% to 93% [26,27].

Skull base and vertebral invasion

Identification of tumor extension to the skull base or prevertebral compartment is important because it frequently indicates inoperability and incurable disease. MR imaging can be used in the assessment of involvement of the prevertebral space. Recently, a larger series of patients with advanced head and neck carcinomas were evaluated

with MR imaging for preservation of the retropharyngeal fat between the tumor and the prevertebral musculature on unenhanced T1-weighted images. This study showed that preservation of this fat plane correctly identified the absence of fixation to the prevertebral muscles in 97.5% of patients [28].

The prevertebral longus muscle complex is evaluated for muscle contour, irregular tumor-muscle interface, T2 hyperintensity, and enhancement. Using these criteria, the accuracy for detection of prevertebral fixation ranges from 56% to 60% [29]. For primary pharyngeal tumors, when there is persistent concern for prevertebral extension, a barium swallow can be obtained to assess whether the posterior pharyngeal wall moves appropriately or whether it is fixed.

Evaluation of adenopathy with an occult primary

In the assessment of pathologic nodes with an unknown primary, knowledge of lymphatic drainage pathways of primary head and neck cancers can be helpful because head and neck cancer has a relatively predictable pattern of metastatic adenopathy based on the site and stage of the primary cancer [Table 1] [30–32]. Nasopharyngeal carcinoma spreads commonly to nasopharyngeal, level II, and level V nodes. Oral cancers, such as floor of mouth and oral tongue cancer, commonly involve level I and II nodes. Cancers of the oropharynx, such as tonsillar and base of tongue carcinoma, typically spread to level II followed by level III nodes. Nodes can be cystic in morphology. The larynx can be divided into three compartments: (1) the supraglottis, (2) the glottis, and (3) the subglottis. Supraglottic larynx has the most abundant lymphatic drainage with nodal metastasis most commonly to level II followed by level III.

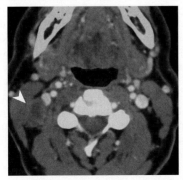

Fig. 14. Contrast-enhanced axial CT scan of the neck shows a necrotic lymph node (*arrowhead*). The fat plane between the lymph node and the adjacent muscle is lost signifying extracapsular spread.

Table 1: Most frequently affected nodal levels by head and neck cancers

Location of cancer	Frequently affected nodal levels
Nasopharynx	Ipsilateral and contralateral levels I and V
Floor of mouth and oral tongue	Ipsilateral levels I and II
Base of tongue and tonsil	Ipsilateral levels II, III and contralateral level II
Soft palate	Ipsilateral and contralateral level II, ipsilateral level III
Supraglottic larynx	Ipsilateral levels II, III, and contralateral level II
Glottis	Ipsilateral levels II and III

The glottis has relatively sparse lymphatic drainage. As a result nodal metastasis is relatively uncommon at the time of presentation of these cancers. The subglottis has intermediate lymphatic drainage, but represents less than 3% of all primary laryngeal cancers.

Paratracheal lymph nodes are frequently associated with laryngeal, thyroid, or lung carcinomas, whereas the presence of supraclavicular and infraclavicular lymphadenopathy may be associated with lung, breast, or gastrointestinal malignancies. The imaging work-up for an unknown primary should include an esophagram and upper gastrointestinal series, and a CT or MR imaging of the chest and abdomen. More recently investigators have been exploring the potential role for positron emission tomography (PET) imaging in this setting. Conventional radiologic techniques usually detect only 25% of primary cancers.

Evolving techniques and contrast agents

Two major pitfalls with conventional MR imaging and CT imaging in assessing for the presence of nodal metastases include misinterpreting benign enlarged, reactive nodes as having metastases, and the inability to detect disease in normal-size nodes that are not necrotic. It is in these nodes in particular that tissue-specific imaging techniques, such as ultrasmall superparamagnetic iron oxide agent (USPIO), can play a significant role in detecting or excluding nodal metastases, improving the diagnostic accuracy of pretherapeutic MR imaging. Advantages of these agents over gadolinium-based contrast agents (or iodine for CT) are that they have a long intravascular half-life (greater than

30 hours) such that delayed imaging 24 to 36 hours after administration continues to show localization of USPIO in the lymph nodes [33]. This gives flexibility in imaging and, in combination with the fact that USPIO causes T1 and T2 shortening (relaxation), provides great potential for their use as an MR imaging contrast agent.

Dextran-coated USPIO accumulates in normal functioning lymph nodes because small iron oxide particles are taken up by macrophages in these nodes. Because of the magnetic susceptibility effects of iron oxide, normal nodes have reduced signal intensity (negative enhancement) on postcontrast T2-weighted spin echo and T2*-weighted gradient echo images [34]. In contrast, because they have reduced phagocytic activity, metastatic nodes remain partially or completely hyperintense on enhanced T2-weighted spin echo and T2*-weighted gradient echo images with a spectrum of observed imaging patterns [35]. Some potential pitfalls of USPIO imaging include obscuration of normal-sized (ie, 4–5 mm) but pathologic lymph nodes because of "blooming" effects on gradient echo imaging of adjacent normal-sized nodes (causing apparent enlargement of nodal size and masking of small nearby metastatic nodes) [35]; reactive follicular hyperplasia, which may mimic metastatic disease because of reduced macrophages-phagocytic activity in these nodes; and necrotic nodes without viable tumor following radiation therapy. The role of USPIO imaging in assessing for recurrent nodal disease in the treated neck requires further prospective investigation.

Tumor recurrence versus treatment changes: a job for positron emission tomography imaging?

One of the most significant challenges facing the radiologist is distinguishing neoplasm from scar following treatment. CT in this regard has limited use because these tissues frequently have overlapping densities, making their distinction difficult. MR imaging can be more sensitive in making this distinction. Postoperative granulation tissue, scar, and fibrosis are dynamic tissues that may have a wide range of intensity and enhancement characteristics. Early scar and granulation tissue tend to be hyperintense on T2-weighted images and enhance following the administration of contrast material, which may make distinction from tumor difficult until growth is demonstrated.

New imaging techniques outside of cross-sectional imaging have focused on the physiologic properties of tumors and tissue characterization, rather than anatomic detail. PET using 2-[F-18] fluoro-2-deoxy-D-glucose (FDG) relies on the metabolic activity of neoplasms relative to adjacent tissues (normal neck soft tissues, scar, fibrosis, inflammatory changes) in positively identifying the presence of tumor [36]. PET imaging may be useful in the detection of unknown primary cancers, in guiding endoscopic biopsies, in evaluating recurrent tumors, and in distinguishing recurrent neoplasm from radiation changes. One of the potential pitfalls of CT and MR imaging is their inability to distinguish treatment changes from recurrent tumor. In general, recurrent neoplasms show significant uptake of FDG compared with fibrotic tissue and radiation-induced changes; however, occasionally, radiation necrosis may demonstrate increased metabolic activity resulting in significant uptake of FDG [36,37]. Furthermore, the timing of FDG PET following irradiation is important in the distinction of radiation changes from tumor. PET performed shortly after radiotherapy may not accurately reflect disease activity, whereas PET acquired several months out may more reliably identify recurrence.

Summary

Clinical palpation for lymph nodes in malignant disease is not highly reliable with a sensitivity of 65% and an accuracy of approximately 75%. Imaging can identify pathologic cervical adenopathy in a significant number of patients with head and neck cancer who have no palpable adenopathy on physical examination. This article reviews nodal classification, drainage patterns of different head and neck cancers, various cross-sectional imaging features of metastatic lymph nodes from head and neck cancer, nodal staging, and certain features like extracapsular spread and carotid and vertebral invasion that the clinician should know because they have therapeutic and prognostic implications. New imaging techniques and the role of FDG PET imaging in recurrent disease are discussed.

References

[1] American cancer society. Cancer facts and figures 2005. Atlanta: American Cancer Society; 2005.

[2] Haberal I, Celik H, Gocmen H, et al. Which is important in the evaluation of metastatic lymph nodes in head and neck cancer: palpation, ultrasonography, or computed tomography? Otolaryngol Head Neck Surg 2004;130:197–201.

[3] Alderson DJ, Jones TM, White SJ, et al. Observer error in the assessment of nodal disease in head and neck cancer. Head Neck 2001;23:739–43.

[4] Atula TS, Varpula MJ, Kurki TJ, et al. Assessment of cervical lymph node status in head and neck cancer patients: palpation, computed tomography and low field magnetic resonance imaging compared with ultrasound-guided fine-needle aspiration cytology. Eur J Radiol 1997;25:152–61.

[5] American Joint Committee on Cancer Staging. American Joint Committee on Cancer Staging manual. 5th edition. Philadelphia: Lippincott Raven; 1997.

[6] Som PM. Lymph nodes. In: Som PM, Curtin HD, editors. Head and neck imaging. 4th edition. St Louis: Mosby; 2003. p. 1865–934.

[7] Yousem DM, Som PM, Hackney DB, et al. Central nodal necrosis and extracapsular neoplastic spread in cervical lymph nodes: MR imaging versus CT. Radiology 1992;182:753–9.

[8] King AD, Tse GM, Ahuja AT, et al. Necrosis in metastatic neck nodes: diagnostic accuracy of CT, MR imaging, and US. Radiology 2004;230: 720–6.

[9] Don DM, Anzai Y, Lufkin RB, et al. Evaluation of cervical lymph node metastases in squamous cell carcinoma of the head and neck. Laryngoscope 1995;105(7 Pt 1):669–74.

[10] Friedman M, Roberts N, Kirshenbaum GL, et al. Nodal size of metastatic squamous cell carcinoma of the neck. Laryngoscope 1993;103:854–6.

[11] Eisenkraft BL, Som PM. The spectrum of benign and malignant etiologies of cervical node calcification. AJR Am J Roentgenol 1999;172:1433–7.

[12] Vassallo P, Wernecke K, Roos N, et al. Differentiation of benign from malignant superficial lymphadenopathy: the role of high-resolution US. Radiology 1992;183:215–20.

[13] Vassallo P, Edel G, Roos N, et al. In-vitro high-resolution ultrasonography of benign and malignant lymph nodes: a sonographic-pathologic correlation. Invest Radiol 1993;28:698–705.

[14] Ying M, Ahuja A, Brook F, et al. Power Doppler sonography of normal cervical lymph nodes. J Ultrasound Med 2000;19:511–7.

[15] van den Brekel MW, Castelijns JA, Stel HV, et al. Modern imaging techniques and ultrasound-guided aspiration cytology for the assessment of neck node metastases: a prospective comparative study. Eur Arch Otorhinolaryngol 1993;250: 11–7.

[16] Chikui T, Yonetsu K, Nakamura T. Multivariate feature analysis of sonographic findings of metastatic cervical lymph nodes: contribution of blood flow features revealed by power Doppler sonography for predicting metastasis. AJNR Am J Neuroradiol 2000;21:561–7.

[17] Sumi M, Ohki M, Nakamura T. Comparison of sonography and CT for differentiating benign from malignant cervical lymph nodes in patients with squamous cell carcinoma of the head and neck. AJR Am J Roentgenol 2001;176:1019–24.

[18] Wu CH, Hsu MM, Chang YL, et al. Vascular pathology of malignant cervical lymphadenopathy: qualitative and quantitative assessment with power Doppler ultrasound. Cancer 1998; 83:1189–96.

[19] Ariji Y, Kimura Y, Hayashi N, et al. Power Doppler sonography of cervical lymph nodes in

patients with head and neck cancer. AJNR Am J Neuroradiol 1998;19:303–7.

[20] Knappe M, Louw M, Gregor RT. Ultrasonography-guided fine-needle aspiration for the assessment of cervical metastases. Arch Otolaryngol Head Neck Surg 2000;126:1091–6.

[21] Baatenburg de Jong RJ, Rongen RJ, Verwoerd CD, et al. Ultrasound-guided fine-needle aspiration biopsy of neck nodes. Arch Otolaryngol Head Neck Surg 1991;117:402–4.

[22] Brasilino de Carvalho M. Quantitative analysis of the extent of extracapsular invasion and its prognostic significance: a prospective study of 170 cases of carcinoma of the larynx and hypopharynx. Head Neck 1998;20:16–21.

[23] Greenberg JS, Fowler R, Gomez J, et al. Extent of extracapsular spread: a critical prognosticator in oral tongue cancer. Cancer 2003;97:1464–70.

[24] Steinkamp HJ, van der Hoeck E, Bock JC, et al. The extracapsular spread of cervical lymph node metastases: the diagnostic value of computed tomography. Rofo Fortschr Geb Rontgenstr Neuen Bildgeb Verfahr 1999;170:457–62.

[25] Steinkamp HJ, Beck A, Werk M, et al. Extracapsular spread of cervical lymph node metastases: diagnostic value of magnetic resonance imaging. Rofo Fortschr Geb Rontgenstr Neuen Bildgeb Verfahr 2002;174:50–5.

[26] Yousem DM, Hatabu H, Hurst RW, et al. Carotid artery invasion by head and neck masses: prediction with MR imaging. Radiology 1995;195:715–20.

[27] Gritzmann N, Grasl MC, Helmer M, et al. Invasion of the carotid artery and jugular vein by lymph node metastases: detection with sonography. AJR Am J Roentgenol 1990;154:411–4.

[28] Hsu WC, Loevner LA, Karpati R, et al. Accuracy of magnetic resonance imaging in predicting absence of fixation of head and neck cancer to the prevertebral space. Head Neck 2005;27:95–100.

[29] Loevner LA, Ott IL, Yousem DM, et al. Neoplastic fixation to the prevertebral compartment by squamous cell carcinoma of the head and neck. AJR Am J Roentgenol 1998;170:1389–94.

[30] Byers RM, Wolf PF, Ballantyne AJ. Rationale for elective modified neck dissection. Head Neck Surg 1988;10:160–7.

[31] Lindberg R. Distribution of cervical lymph node metastasis from squamous cell carcinoma of the upper respiratory and digestive tracts. Cancer 1972;29:1446–9.

[32] Mukherji SK, Armao D, Joshi VM. Cervical nodal metastases in squamous cell carcinoma of the head and neck: what to expect. Head Neck 2001;23:995–1005.

[33] Hudgins PA, Anzai Y, Morris MR, et al. Ferumoxtran-10, a superparamagnetic iron oxide as a magnetic resonance enhancement agent for imaging lymph nodes: a phase 2 dose study. AJNR Am J Neuroradiol 2002;23:649–56.

[34] Mack MG, Balzer JO, Straub R, et al. Superparamagnetic iron oxide-enhanced MR imaging of head and neck lymph nodes. Radiology 2002;222:239–44.

[35] Sigal R, Vogl T, Casselman J, et al. Lymph node metastases from head and neck squamous cell carcinoma: MR imaging with ultrasmall superparamagnetic iron oxide particles (Sinerem MR). Results of a phase-III multicenter clinical trial. Eur Radiol 2002;12:1104–13.

[36] Hanasono MM, Kunda LD, Segall GM, et al. Uses and limitations of FDG positron emission tomography in patients with head and neck cancer. Laryngoscope 1999;109:880–5.

[37] McCollum AD, Burrell SC, Haddad RI, et al. Positron emission tomography with 18F-fluorodeoxyglucose to predict pathologic response after induction chemotherapy and definitive chemoradiotherapy in head and neck cancer. Head Neck 2004;26:890–6.

ELSEVIER SAUNDERS

RADIOLOGIC
CLINICS
OF NORTH AMERICA

Radiol Clin N Am 44 (2006) 111–133

MR Imaging of Epilepsy: Strategies for Successful Interpretation

Venkatramana R. Vattipally, MD, Richard A. Bronen, MD*

The first half of this article is devoted to providing an introduction and overview for MR imaging of epilepsy. Several MR imaging epilepsy topics will be discussed in great detail in separate articles, such as hippocampal sclerosis, developmental disorders, and functional MR imaging. The remainder of this review will discuss strategies for successful interpretation of MR images from the seizure patient and how to avoid potential pitfalls.

Overview of epilepsy

Epilepsy is a chronic, neurologic disorder characterized by spontaneous, recurrent seizures. Seizures are caused by excessive and abnormal electrical discharges from the cortical neurons.

The epilepsies and epilepsy syndromes are broadly classified into generalized and focal [1]. Partial (focal) seizures originate from a localized area of the brain, whereas generalized seizures originate simultaneously from both cerebral hemispheres. Partial seizures are further subdivided into simple partial, without loss of any consciousness, and complex partial, with loss of consciousness. Partial seizures can spread from one area to another and become secondarily generalized seizures. Though most patients with epilepsy caused by generalized seizures respond to antiepileptic drugs, 30% of those with partial seizures are resistant to antiepileptic drugs [2,3]. In these patients, surgical resection of the brain region provoking seizures is often the only effective treatment. Medically refractory epilepsy is a social, economic, and medical burden not only to the affected individual but also the community in general. Thus, the classification of seizures has prognostic and therapeutic values that help in the improved management and care of patients with epilepsy.

Epilepsy is a common disorder, with a prevalence of 0.4% to 1% of the population [4–6]. MR imaging is an excellent tool for detecting anatomic substrates that underlie regional brain epileptogenesis, but this potential is dependent on the particular population that is being examined. In a study of 300 consecutive patients presenting with first seizure, an epileptogenic lesion was identified by MR imaging in

This article was originally published in *Neuroimaging Clinics of North America* 14:349–72, 2004.
Yale University School of Medicine, New Haven, CT, USA
* Corresponding author. Yale University School of Medicine, 333 Cedar Street, New Haven, CT 06510.
E-mail address: richard.bronen@yale.edu (R.A. Bronen).

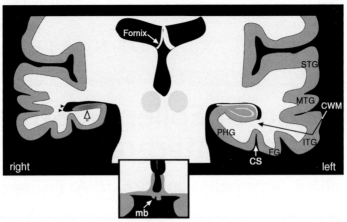

Fig. 1. Coronal T1-weighted diagram of hippocampal sclerosis. Hippocampal atrophy (*open arrow*), the primary finding of hippocampal sclerosis, is demonstrated on the right (the other primary finding of abnormal increased T2 signal intensity is not depicted). The right hippocampus shows loss of the normal alternating gray and white matter internal architecture (compare with the normal left hippocampus). Secondary MR findings of mesial temporal sclerosis include ipsilateral atrophy of the temporal lobe, parahippocampal white matter (PHG), fornix, and mammilary body (mb). The *insert* represents the mammilary body on a more anterior image. Ipsilateral temporal horn dilatation (*arrowheads*) and atrophy of the white matter (CWM) between the hippocampus and gray matter overlying the collateral sulcus (CS) is also depicted. (*From* Bronen RA. MR of mesial temporal sclerosis: how much is enough? AJNR Am J Neuroradiol 1998;19(1):15–8; with permission.)

14% (38/263) [7]. In another study, MR imaging detected etiologically relevant structural abnormalities in 12.7% (62/388) of children with newly diagnosed epilepsy [8]. In intractable epilepsy, the overall sensitivity of MR imaging in identifying substrates is in the range of 82% to 86% [9,10]. In a study of 117 patients with intractable epilepsy who underwent surgery, the sensitivities of CT and MR imaging in detecting structural abnormalities were 32% (35/109) and 95% (104/109) respectively [9]. However, MR imaging is of little benefit in those with idiopathic generalized epilepsy. One study found no structural abnormalities in subjects with idiopathic generalized epilepsy or benign rolandic epilepsy [7]. Based on these and other studies, published guidelines indicate that MR imaging must always be performed in the nonemergent setting in patients with epilepsy, with the exception of primary idiopathic generalized epilepsy. CT still has a role in the initial evaluation of seizures when associated with focal neurologic changes, fever, trauma, or in an emergency setting [11–14].

Role of MR imaging

The main purpose of neuroimaging in epilepsy patients is to identify underlying structural abnormalities that require specific treatment (ie, sur-

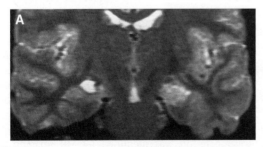
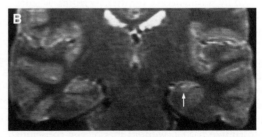

Fig. 2. Hippocampal sclerosis and choroidal fissure cyst. Coronal T2-weighted image (*A*) shows a hyperintense lesion adjacent to the right hippocampus, which did not match a left temporal lobe clinical seizure source. If one focused solely on this obvious lesion, one would neglect the small hyperintense left hippocampus (*arrow*), which was surgically proven to represent hippocampal sclerosis (*B*). The right-sided lesion was a choroidal fissure cyst. It was isointense to CSF on all pulse sequences and located in choroidal fissure above the hippocampus. (*From* Bronen RA, Cheung G, Charles JT, et al. Imaging findings in hippocampal sclerosis: correlation with pathology. AJNR Am J Neuroradiol 1991;12(5):933–40; with permission.)

gery in most instances) and also to aid in formulating a syndromic or etiologic diagnosis. With recent advances in techniques, previously undetectable subtle structural abnormalities are now routinely demonstrated by MR imaging. As compared with CT, MR imaging—with its higher sensitivity, better spatial resolution, excellent soft tissue contrast, multiplanar imaging capability, and lack of ionizing radiation—emerged as primary modality of choice in the evaluation of patients with epilepsy.

In epilepsy surgery, MR plays a crucial role not only in identifying the anatomic location of a substrate but also in depicting the relationship of the substrate to the eloquent regions of the brain (eg, cortices involved with motor, speech, or memory function). Correlation and concordance of MR imaging identified substrate with clinical and electrophysiologic data is essential to avoid false positive localization of the epileptogenic substrate [15]. Concordance of noninvasive electrophysiologic data with MR may obviate the need for invasive electroencephalographic monitoring.

Postoperative MR imaging may identify the complications of surgery as well as causes for the surgical treatment failure, such as residual/recurrent lesion. MR imaging can also prognosticate the post-

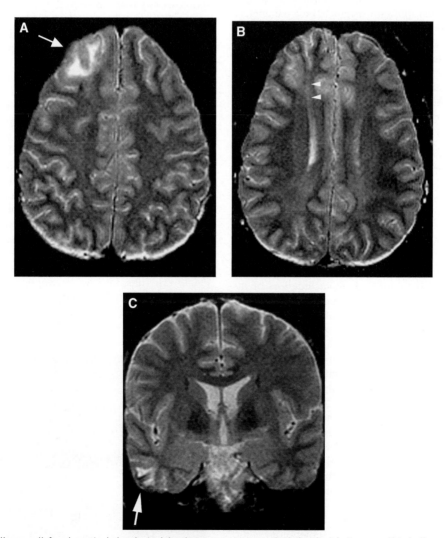

Fig. 3. Balloon cell focal cortical dysplasia (also known type II cortical dysplasia). Because this balloon cell focal cortical dysplastic lesion (*A, B*) has hyperintense signal changes in the subcortical white matter (*A*) on long TR images, it may be confused with a neoplasm (*C*). However, unlike tumors, balloon cell focal cortical dysplasia is associated with cortical thickening (compare the thickened cortex in (*A*) to the normal cortex in (*C*) (*arrows*). A radial band (*arrowheads* in *B*) in this case of dysplasia also helps to distinguish this from neoplasm. (*From* Bronen RA, Vives KP, Kim JH, et al. Focal cortical dysplasia of Taylor balloon cell subtype: MR differentiation from low-grade tumors. AJNR Am J Neuroradiol 1997;18(6):1141–51; with permission.)

operative seizure control of epileptogenic substrates. Postoperative seizure control depends on the identification of the substrate by MR imaging and the characteristics of the MR abnormality [16].

MR imaging of epileptogenic substrates

Focal epilepsy can be categorized into the following five groups or substrates: (1) hippocampal sclerosis, (2) malformations of cortical development, (3) neoplasms, (4) vascular abnormalities, and (5) gliosis and miscellaneous abnormalities [17]. Each substrate can be defined by a set of characteristic parameters, which unite all abnormalities within each particular substrate category. These parameters include etiology, mechanism of action, treatment options, and postoperative outcome. Because hippocampal sclerosis and developmental abnormalities are discussed separately, here the authors concentrate on the vascular, neoplastic, gliosis, and miscellaneous substrates, with brief references to hippocampal sclerosis and developmental disorders.

Hippocampal sclerosis

Hippocampal sclerosis is the most common epileptogenic substrate seen throughout various surgical epilepsy series. Anterior temporal lobectomy cures the epilepsy in 67% of patients with hippocampal sclerosis [18]. Hippocampal sclerosis is characterized by neuronal loss and gliosis [19,20]. The most important MR findings in hippocampal sclerosis are atrophy and abnormal T2 signal [**Figs. 1 and 2**] [20–22]. Other minor findings include loss of internal architecture, loss of hippocampal head interdigitations [23], atrophy of ipsilateral mammilary body and fornix [24], dilatation of the ipsilateral temporal horn, volume loss of the temporal lobe, and atrophy of the collateral white matter between the hippocampus and collateral sulcus [25]. The sensitivity of MR in detecting hippocampal sclerosis by qualitative assessment is in the range of 80% to 90%, and by quantitative methods, the sensitivity climbs to 90% to 95% in surgical intractable epilepsy patients [26–28]. Bilateral hippocampal atrophy without obvious signal changes on long TR images, which occurs in 10% to 20% of cases, can be diagnosed by hippocampal volumetry and T2 relaxometry. Hippocampal volumetry and T2 relaxometry can also be useful in lateralizing the epileptogenic lesion [29,30]. Dual pathology is the coexistence of hippocampal sclerosis with another epileptogenic substrate. It occurs in 8% to 22% of surgical epilepsy patients [31]. The most common substrate visualized along with hippocampal sclerosis is cortical dysgenesis. Lesionectomy and hippocampectomy may improve the surgical success in

controlling seizures in patients with dual pathology [32,33].

Malformations of cortical development

Developmental malformations are increasingly recognized by MR imaging as causes of epilepsy in children and young adults. At the present time, developmental malformations constitute 10% to 50% of pediatric epilepsy cases being evaluated for surgery and 4% to 25% of adult cases [34–36]. The most widely used classification of malformations of cortical development (MCD) divides these entities into four categories: (1) malformations due to abnormal neuronal and glial proliferation or apoptosis, (2) malformations due to abnormal neuronal migration [**Figs. 3 and 4**], (3) malformations due to abnormal cortical organization [**Fig. 5**], and (4) malformations of cortical development, not otherwise classified [37].

MR imaging findings in MCD include cortical thickening, morphologic abnormalities in sulci and gyri, blurring of gray/white matter junction, areas of T2 prolongation in the cortex or subjacent white matter with/without extension toward the ventricles, heterotopic gray matter [21,38], and cerebral spinal fluid (CSF) clefts and cortical dimple [Box 1] [39]. Many developmental malformations are intrinsically epileptogenic. It is important to be aware that the extent of the epileptogenic zone may be more extensive than the structural abnormalities visible on MR images and that epileptogenic zone may not correlate directly to the malformation but may be at a distance from the malformation [34,40,41]. Thus, invasive electrophysiologic studies (ie, subdural and depth electrodes) are usually considered in the presurgical evaluation of these

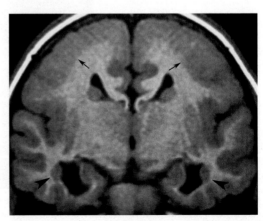

Fig. 4. Pachygyria and heteropia. T1-weighted coronal image demonstrates pachygyria with macrogyria, cortical thickening, and loss of gray-white distinction (*arrows*) as well as heterotopia (*arrowheads*) and agenesis of corpus callosum.

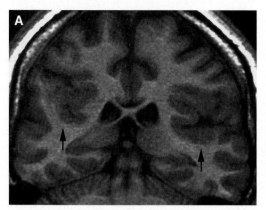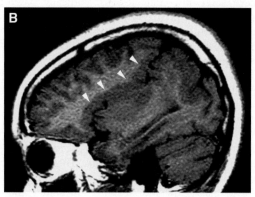

Fig. 5. Polymicrogyria. (*A*) Coronal T1-weighted imaging shows an abnormal sylvian fissure morphology associated with marked cortical thickening (*arrows*). The sagittal image (*B*) demonstrates an abnormal sylvian fissure (*arrowheads*), which has become contiguous with the central sulcus.

malformations [35,42]. Because many of these malformations may be subtle, high-resolution imaging with good gray-white matter differentiating sequences and a systemic approach in interpretation of images are essential for identification and characterization of these substrates [43].

Neoplasms

Brain tumors constitute 2% to 4% of epileptogenic substrates in the general epilepsy population. MR imaging has a sensitivity of nearly 100% in detecting neoplastic lesions, 68% of which are located in temporal lobes in epilepsy patients [9]. Epileptogenic neoplasms associated with chronic epilepsy are located near the cortex in 90% of patients, in the temporal lobe in 68%, and not usually associated with mass effect or vasogenic edema [44]. These focal lesions are often associated with calvarial remodeling corresponding with their indolent nature and chronic presence. The epileptogenic focus is usually localized in the surrounding brain parenchyma, but in some cases, such as hypothalamic

hamartomas, the neoplasm has intrinsic epileptogenicity. Complete resection of the neoplasm and overlying cortex results in successful control of seizures in most cases; partial resection of tumor can result in improvement in quality of life by decrease in the frequency of seizures [44,45].

Various neoplasms are found in patients with seizures, including low-grade astrocytic tumors, ganglioglioma, dysembryoplastic neuroepithelial tumor (DNET), oligodendroglioma, pleomorphic xanthoastrocytoma, and cerebral metastasis. Most neoplasms are hypointense on T1-weighted images and hyperintense on T2-weighted images. It is often difficult to predict tumor histology in an individual from the MR imaging findings, although certain characteristics tend to be associated with some types of tumors.

Astrocytomas

Astrocytomas have nonspecific imaging features. As a group, the fibrillary subtype (WHO grade 2) is often a low-grade, ill-defined infiltrative tumor that usually does not enhance with contrast, whereas pilocytic astrocytomas are well-defined lesions that usually enhance with contrast [45,46].

Oligodendroglioma

Oligodendroglioma is a slow-growing, peripherally located lesion commonly seen in the frontal or frontotemporal cortex. On MR imaging, these tumors may appear as cortical-based lesions in the frontal lobe with calcifications and adjacent calvarial changes. Contrast enhancement is variable.

Ganglioglioma

Ganglioglioma is commonly seen in temporal lobe, usually occurring in patients less than 30 years old (peak age is 10 to 20 years). These are benign,

---

Box 1: Imaging features of cortical dysgenesis

Cortical thickening
Blurring of gray-white junction
Irregularity of gray-white junction
Macrogyria
Mini-gyria (polymicrogyria)
Paucity of gyri
Sulcal cleft and cortical dimple
Sulcal morphologic changes
Radial bands of hyperintensity
Transmantle gray matter
Gray matter heterotopia
Band heterotopia

mixed solid and cystic lesions, cortically based with minimal or no mass effect or edema. Calcification is often present. Contrast enhancement is variable [47,48]. The combination of calcification and cysts in a cortically based lesion in a patient with seizures should make the practitioner consider this diagnosis.

Dysembryoplastic neuroepithelial tumors

DNETs are benign, low-grade, multicystic, and multinodular cortical-based tumors predominantly seen in children and young adults. These lesions may be associated with calvarial remodeling or cortical dysplasia. The MR imaging appearance and contrast enhancement is variable and nonspecific, unless the imaging features present as a multicystic cortically based tumor [Fig. 6] [46,47].

Pleomorphic xanthoastrocytomas

Pleomorphic xanthoastrocytomas are peripherally located (adjacent to the leptomeninges) cystic lesions with enhancing mural nodule. Involvement of the leptomeninges is the characteristic feature of this tumor. Prognosis is good after surgical resection; however, local recurrence and malignant transformation can occur in these tumors [46,47].

Vascular malformations

Vascular malformations constitute 5% of epileptogenic substrates in the generality of epilepsy patients. Arteriovenous malformations (AVMs) and cavernous malformations (also known as cavernomas or cavernous hemangiomas) are the most common vascular malformations causing seizures in epilepsy patients. The sensitivity of MR imaging is close to 100% in detecting these malformations [44].

Arteriovenous malformations

AVMs are congenital, developmental anomalies of blood vessels. AVMs consist of a tangle of blood vessels lacking intervening capillary network and leading to direct arteriovenous shunting of blood. Thrombosis, calcification, hemorrhage, and fibrosis are common secondary changes in these lesions. The possible mechanisms for seizure generation include (1) focal cerebral ischemia from steal phenomena due to arteriovenous shunting, and (2) gliosis and hemosiderin deposition from subclinical hemorrhage in the brain parenchyma [45]. T1- and T2-weighted images demonstrate serpiginous flow voids with areas of T2 prolongation in the adjoining brain parenchyma. Surgical resection of the AVM is effective in controlling seizures in patients with epilepsy [49].

Cavernous malformations

Cavernous malformations are composed of well-circumscribed vascular spaces containing blood in various stages of evolution. The absence of any intervening neural tissue within the lesion is the hallmark of this lesion. From 15% to 54% of these lesions are multiple, and 50% to 80% of multiple lesions occur on a familial basis [50]. The typical MR appearance of a cavernous malformation is popcorn-like with a heterogeneous hyperintense signal centrally on all pulse sequences, surrounded by a rim of low signal intensity from hemosiderin [Fig. 7]. Because hemosiderin results in magnetic susceptibility artifacts (which are visualized as signal voids on MR images), sequences that are more affected by magnetic susceptibility artifacts will tend to have the greatest sensitivity for detecting small cavernomas. Thus, gradient echo images have a much higher sensitivity when compared with conventional or fast spin echo sequences. Though

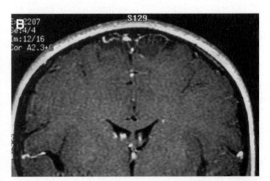

Fig. 6. Dysembryoplastic neuroepithelial tumor. Coronal proton density-weighted image (*A*) and postcontrast (*B*) images demonstrate a peripherally based lesion (*arrow*) with trabeculated enhancement. Based solely on these images, it appears that the lesion is extra-axial because gray matter can be seen surrounding the lesion, especially in (*A*). However, it is not uncommon for an intra-axial neoplasm causing chronic epilepsy to appear extra-axial because it is situated within or replaces the cortex and has the appearance of being outside the cortex in some cross-sectional planes. Thin section imaging allowed visualization of the multicystic nature of this lesion on the enhanced image (*B*).

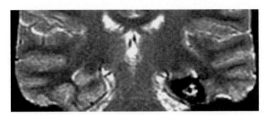

Fig. 7. Cavernous malformation. Coronal T2-weighted image with a temporal lobe lesion. The central hyperintense signal intensity (due to chronic blood products, methemoglobin) surrounded by a rim of signal void (due to hemosiderin) is typical of an occult vascular malformation, which is usually the result of a cavernous malformation, as in this case.

MR imaging has high sensitivity in detecting these lesions, it cannot reliably differentiate between a cavernous hemangioma, a partially thrombosed AVM, or a hemorrhagic metastatic lesion [44]. However, in a patient with epilepsy and typical MR imaging popcorn lesion with a hemosiderin ring, the most likely diagnosis is cavernous malformation.

Developmental venous malformations are discussed in the normal variant section that follows.

Gliosis and miscellaneous abnormalities

A number of disparate entities that are associated with intractable epilepsy have certain histologic findings, with gliosis (and neuronal loss) in common. Gliosis is the end result of various focal and diffuse central nervous system injuries. Examples include trauma, infection, and infarctions, which may be focal or diffuse. Stroke is a common cause of epilepsy in the elderly population [51]. Rasmussen's encephalitis, perinatal insults, and Sturge-Weber syndrome are examples of diffuse entities, which may involve an entire cerebral hemisphere and lead to atrophy of that hemisphere. MR imaging findings of gliosis are nonspecific, consisting of hyperintense changes on long TR sequences and hypointense signal intensity on T1-weighted images, which may be associated with volume loss, encephalomalacia, sulcal widening, and ventricular enlargement. Some of the more important epileptogenic entities in this gliosis and miscellaneous category will be discussed in detail.

Prenatal, perinatal, and postnatal insults

Diffuse and focal destructive lesions of the brain constitute a major group of pathologic processes in children presenting with seizures [52]. The appearance of these lesions depends on the timing of the insults to the brain.

Early injury to the brain of the developing fetus (less than 6 months) leads to the formation of smooth-walled porencephalic cavities with minimal or no glial reaction in the surrounding brain parenchyma [53]. These porencephalic cavities are commonly located in perisylvian regions and are filled with CSF and may communicate with the ventricles, subarachnoid space, or both. Porencephaly is associated with increased incidence of hippocampal sclerosis ipsilateral to the porencephalic cavity, or bilateral [52].

Brain injury occurring in the perinatal or postnatal period leads to a pattern of encephalomalacia or ulegyria. Encephalomalacia (diffuse or focal) results from late gestational, perinatal, and postnatal injuries to the brain. Encephalomalacia results in multiple, irregular cystic cavities with prominent astrocytic proliferation [Fig. 8] [53]. Ulegyria, also a result of perinatal insult to the brain, is commonly seen in the parieto-occipital region. It is characterized by destruction of the gray matter in the depths of the sulci, sparing the crowns of gyral convolutions [54]. MR imaging is useful not only in identifying these lesions and defining their extent in surgically fit patients but also in diagnosing periventricular leucomalacia and multicystic encephalomalacia.

Posttraumatic epilepsy

Posttraumatic epilepsy may be considered a specialized form of postnatal injury epilepsy. The overall risk of seizures is in the range of 1.8% to 5% for civilian injuries, but can be as high as 53% for war injuries [55]. In closed head injuries, the most common sites of injury are along the inferior anterior regions of the brain because of irregularities of the skull base at these locations—the orbital surfaces of the frontal lobe, the undersurface of the temporal lobe, the frontal pole, and the tempo-

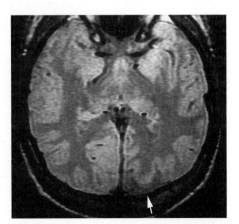

Fig. 8. Gliotic scar. This region of encephalomalacia and gliosis (*arrow*) appears as a widened CSF space on this proton density-weighed image. Surgical removal cured the seizures. (*From* Bronen RA, Fulbright RK, Kim JH, et al. A systematic approach for interpreting MR images of the seizure patient. AJR Am J Roentgenol 1997;169(1):241–7; with permission.)

ral pole. These traumatic shearing injuries of the brain, or contusions, are often associated with hemorrhage, which eventually results in hemosiderin deposition and reparative gliotic changes [56]. Hemosiderin and gliosis are known to be involved in seizure generation/propagation [57].

Risk factors for late posttraumatic epilepsy include (1) early posttraumatic seizures, (2) severe initial brain injury (loss of consciousness or amnesia for more than 24 hours), (3) complex depressed skull fracture, (4) subdural hematoma, (5) penetrating injury, (6) intracranial hemorrhage, (7) brain contusion, and (8) age over 65 years [55,58]. Depressed skull fractures, intracerebral hematoma and subdural hematoma carry a risk of 25% for

developing post traumatic seizures [58]. MR imaging is an effective modality for demonstrating diffuse axonal injury, intracerebral hematoma, subdural hematoma, contusions, and gliosis. Because hemosiderin is not completely removed from the brain, MR imaging can detect evidence of old hemorrhagic lesions. Thus, MR imaging plays a role in the management of patients with trauma and may be a useful tool in predicting the prognosis for the patient in the long run.

Infections

Seizures can be an early clinical sign in bacterial, viral, fungal, mycobacterial, and parasitic infections. In the acute phase, the seizures may be re-

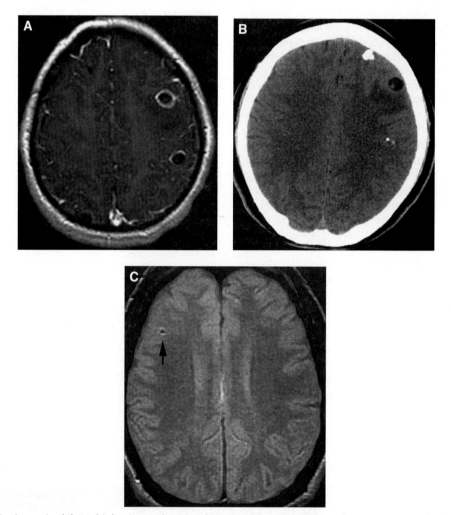

Fig. 9. Cysticercosis. (*A*) Multiple ring enhancing lesions with surrounding edema represent the inflammatory reactive stage of cysticercosis on this contrast enhanced T1-weighted axial image. Corresponding CT scan (*B*) shows calcification of these lesions. In a different patient, the only MR abnormality was the punctate signal void (*arrow*) in the right frontal lobe on this proton density-weighted image (*C*). This was surgically proven to represent a calcified granuloma due to cysticercosis that caused chronic epilepsy. (**Fig. 9***C from* Bronen RA, Fulbright RK, Kim JH, et al. A systematic approach for interpreting MR images of the seizure patient. AJR Am J Roentgenol 1997;169(1):241–7; with permission.)

lated to the host's inflammatory response, and may be due to gliotic changes in the chronic phase. With the recent advances in imaging and increase in the immigrant population, tuberculosis and neurocysticercosis are increasingly documented as the most common infections, with seizure presentation in developed and developing countries.

Neurocysticercosis results from infestation with larval form of pig tapeworm *Taenia solium.* Neurocysticercosis can be seen in parenchyma, ventricles, subarachnoid spaces, or a combination of these. Seizures are the result of the inflammatory response to the dying and degenerating parasite.

In the active parenchymal form, cysticercosis is visualized on MR images as thin-walled nonenhancing cystic lesions isointense to CSF on all pulse sequences. Within the cyst, an eccentrically located scolex may be seen, which usually enhances. In the inactive parenchymal or dying form, with increasing inflammatory changes from the host response, the cyst wall thickens and enhances after contrast administration. Vasogenic edema is usually seen in the adjoining brain parenchyma, and the fluid in the cyst also increases in signal on T1-weighted images. With further progression of inflammatory changes, the cystic lesion is replaced by granuloma, seen on MR imaging as an enhancing nodule. After the death of the larvae, the cysts and scolices are replaced by dense calcification, which are visualized as signal voids on gradient echo images as a result of susceptibility artifacts [59]. Most of the calcified lesions are located at the gray/white matter junction [Fig. 9].

Tuberculosis is a chronic granulomatous infection caused by *Mycobacterium.* It is characterized by caseous central necrosis and the presence of multi-nucleated giant cells in the granuloma. Risk factors include elderly age, poverty, human immunodeficiency virus (HIV), immunosuppression, and lymphoma. Incidence of central nervous system tuberculosis in the HIV-negative pulmonary tuberculosis population is 2%, and 19% in the HIV-positive pulmonary tuberculosis patients [60]. Central nervous system tuberculosis can involve the meninges and brain parenchyma, and the leptomeningeal version can cause hydrocephalus, neuropathies, arthritis, and deep gray matter infarction.

Parenchymal tuberculomas can be single or multiple. The MR imaging findings are nonspecific and depend on the host hypersensitivity reaction to the bacillus. The amount of host hypersensitivity reaction predicts the amount of inflammatory cells, gliosis, and free radical deposition in the granuloma. The noncaseating tuberculoma can be seen as an iso- to hypointense lesion on T1-weighted images and as a variable signal intensity lesion on T2-weighted images, with surrounding edema. The granuloma enhances homogenously after contrast administration. Caseating granulomas are hypo- to isointense on T1-weighted images and hypointense to brain parenchyma on T2-weighted images, enhancing in a ring-like manner. Small lesions detected by MR imaging are more amenable to medical treatment, and thus MR imaging can have a prognostic value by identifying and determining their size [60].

Rasmussen's encephalitis

Rasmussen's encephalitis is chronic encephalitis characterized by partial motor seizures and progressive neurologic and cognitive deterioration [54,61,62]. It usually affects one cerebral hemisphere, which later becomes atrophic. Most cases are seen in children, though some are also reported in adolescents and adults.

The disease progresses through three phases. In the initial prodromal phase, the patient presents with few partial motor seizures. The second phase, the acute stage, is characterized by an increase in frequency of partial motor seizures. In the last or residual phase, there are permanent and stable neurologic deficits [61]. MR imaging findings in the acute phase include areas of T2 prolongation in the cortex and subcortical white matter, usually starting in the frontoinsular region and extending to other parts of the brain. These signal changes in the cortex and subcortical white matter can be fleeting—changing in size and location over time. Cortical atrophy with ventricular enlargement and caudate nucleus atrophy can be seen as the disease progresses [61]. In late stages of this disorder, atrophy of the entire cerebral hemisphere with

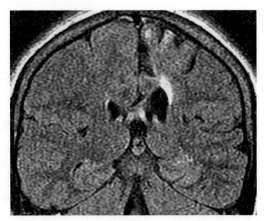

Fig. 10. Rasmussen's encephalitis. Coronal FLAIR image demonstrates encephalomalacia in the left frontoparietal region with abnormal signal in the left paracentral lobule and exvacuo dilatation of the left lateral ventricle in a patient with pathologically proven Rasmussen's encephalitis.

hemi-atrophy of the ipsilateral brain stem may be seen, and when associated with contralateral cerebellar diaschis is due to degeneration of cortico-pontocerebellar fibers [Fig. 10].

Sturge-Weber syndrome

Sturge-Weber syndrome is a sporadic, congenital neurocutaneous syndrome characterized by the association of ipsilateral facial angioma in the distribution of the trigeminal nerve with angiomatosis of the leptomeninges. Clinically, patients present with facial angioma, intractable seizures, hemiparesis, hemianopsia, and mental retardation. A dysgenetic venous system is responsible for most of the imaging and clinical findings in these patients.

Intractable epilepsy is the earliest and most common clinical presentation in these patients. MR can demonstrate the structural abnormalities in the brain, which include (1) pial angiomata in the parietal occipital region on post–contrast-enhanced images, (2) cortical calcifications subjacent to the cortex and white matter in the parieto-occipital region, which are depicted as signal voids or hypointense curvilinear structures, (3) enlarged choroid plexus, especially on postcontrast enhanced images, (4) atrophy of the ipsilateral cerebral hemisphere (angioma side), and (5) enlarged and elongated globe of the eye [Fig. 11] [63]. The pial angioma is believed to be due to the persistence of embryonic vasculature. It is generally accepted

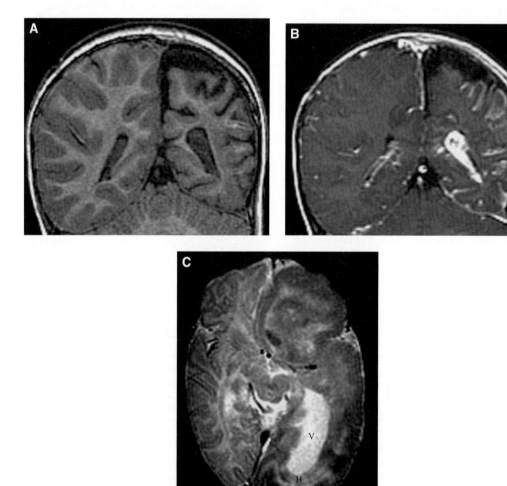

Fig. 11. Hemiatrophy and hemisphere asymmetry. (*A*) T1-weighted coronal image demonstrates asymmetry of the hemispheres. Because the CSF spaces and ventricle are larger ipsilateral to the smaller hemisphere, this represents hemiatrophy. Based solely on this image, it is difficult to distinguish the cause of the hemiatrophy. However, in this case of Sturge-Weber syndrome, a contrast-enhanced scan (*B*) is helpful, depicting marked enhancement along the pial surface and ipsilateral choroidal plexus. (*C*) Hemimegalencephaly is also associated with hemisphere and ventricular asymmetry, but the larger ventricle (V) is ipsilateral to the larger hemisphere. This entity is also associated with heterotopias (H) and cortical thickening (C).

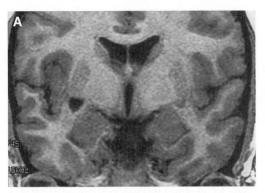

Fig. 12. Subcapsular Virchow Robbin spaces. This subcapsular lesion is isointense to CSF on coronal T1-weighted (A) and T2-weighted (B) images. This unilateral lesion may give one pause, but Virchow Robbin spaces in this location inferior to the basal ganglia are common, although they are usually bilateral and smaller in size.

that the calcifications in the cortex and the subjacent white matter are caused by chronic ischemia, and enlarged choroids plexus is the result of shunted venous drainage from the cerebral hemisphere to the choroids plexus. Other associated features include prominent and enlarged subependymal and medullary veins (due to dysgenetic superficial venous system) and secondary signs of cerebral atrophy, which include dilated paranasal sinuses, mastoid air cells, and thickened calvarium.

Imaging issues: strategies for successful interpretation

Successful MR imaging of the seizure patient can be more demanding than brain imaging of other patients because the abnormalities may be subtle and not easily visualized with routine brain imaging sequences. This necessitates dedicated imaging sequences, a high index of suspicion, and careful review of imaging studies. Some abnormalities present as minor asymmetries of brain structure, so practitioners must be able to differentiate normal variations from pathologic conditions. This section discusses some practical issues with respect to MR imaging of epilepsy: normal anatomic and imaging variations, an approach to image interpretation, differential diagnosis, and imaging protocol.

Normal variations

CSF or cystlike structures are frequently present in healthy individuals. The following CSF structures have no relationship to epilepsy in general and must be differentiated from pathologic conditions. One correlative MR-histologic study found cysts and punctate foci of T2 signal changes in 17% (n = 17) of patients with surgical intractable epilepsy [9]. Arachnoid cysts and choroidal fissure cysts are isointense to CSF on all pulse sequences [see Fig. 2]

[64]. Perivascular Virchow-Robbin spaces are commonly visualized in patients with seizures because the dedicated imaging sequences allow for better detail than routine sequences. Asymmetric large Virchow-Robbin spaces in the region of the anterior perforated substance and subcapsular region may give pause to the uninitiated, but are common occurrences [Fig. 12]. Virchow-Robbin spaces in the subinsular zone (ie, between the extreme and external capsules) may appear lesion-like on T2-weighted fast spin echo sequences [Fig. 13] [65]. However, because Virchow-Robbin spaces represent CSF in perivascular space, these "anomalies" are always isointense to CSF. Feather-like configurations may be detected on T2-weighted images.

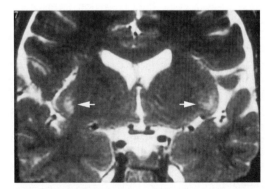

Fig. 13. Subinsular Virchow Robbin spaces. The hyperintense signals (arrows) in the extreme and external capsules on this T2-weighted coronal image are caused by Virchow Robbin spaces. Their true nature can be recognized by noting the feathered configuration, typical location, and isointensity to CSF on all sequences. (From Song CJ, Kim JH, Kier EL, Bronen RA. MR and histology of subinsular T2-weighted bright spots: Virchow-Robbin spaces of the extreme capsule and insula cortex. Radiology 2000;214:671–7; with permission.).

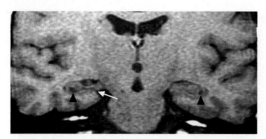

Fig. 14. Cyst of hippocampal sulcal remnant. A common variation occurs when the lateral portion of the hippocampal sulcus (*arrow*) does not normally involute and instead forms a hippocampal sulcal remnant cyst (*arrowheads*). (*From* Bronen RA, Cheung G. MRI of the normal hippocampus. Magn Reson Imaging 1991; 9(4):497–500; with permission.)

Partial volume effects with the brain may lead to mild hypointense signal intensity compared with brain on T1-weighted images rather than the more marked hypointensity of CSF that is found in the ventricles. Punctate or linear enhancement within the center of these represents the vasculature and confirms the diagnosis (but there should be no other enhancement associated with these). Similar findings may be found along the subcortical zone of the anterior temporal lobe cortex, which also represents Virchow-Robbin spaces (Zhang W et al, unpublished data) and these again need to be distinguished from pathologic conditions. A normal variant seen in 10% to 15% of the normal population is the cyst of hippocampal sulcal. The hippocampal sulcus, located between the cornu ammonis and dentate gyrus, normally involutes in utero. In some cases, a cystic fluid collection forms if the lateral potion of the sulcus fails to involute. This cyst is located in the hippocampus itself, between dentate gyrus and cornua ammonis and is isointense to CSF in all pulse sequences [Fig. 14]. It does not demonstrate any contrast enhancement [66,67]. The uncal recess or anterior-most portion of the temporal horn is asymmetric in 60% of epilepsy patients as well as healthy individuals and has no relationship to epileptogenic zone (Messinger JM, Bronen RA, Kier EL, unpublished data), and is easily misinterpreted by those unfamiliar with this finding [Fig. 15].

Isolated developmental venous malformations, also known as venous angiomas or developmental venous anomalies, have not been implicated in epileptogenesis [68,69]. However, venous anomalies are not infrequently found in conjunction with other abnormalities that have been linked to epilepsy, such as cavernous malformations and malformations of cortical development (such as the perisylvian polymicrogyria and other polymicrogyrial syndromes).

Detection of cortical abnormalities underlying malformations of cortical development can be difficult, and practitioners need to be cognizant about the normal variants of gyral and sulcal configurations. The cortex adjoining the superior temporal sulcus on the right side is usually slightly thicker than that of the left side (Zhang W, Schultz R, Bronen RA, unpublished data) and can be misinterpreted as a region of dysplasia. Similarly, the gyri surrounding the calcarine sulcus usually indents the occipital horn (in an area known as the calcar avis), giving rise to the appearance of thickened gyri, which can be misinterpreted as cortical dysplasia if it is asymmetric [70]. Because of the normal undulations of the cortex, there are frequently brain regions with the appearance of cortical thickening on cross-sectional images, if the gyrus is parallel to cross-sectional plane. Dysplasia can be distinguished from this normal finding by observing cortical thickening on multiple images (usually at least three contiguous this section images) or confirming that cortical thickening is present in another plane [Fig. 16]. The signal intensity of gray and white matter in the immature myelinated infant can be confusing and lead to misinterpretations. For instance, the myelinated optic radiation surrounded by unmyelinated white matter could be mistaken for gray matter and labeled as band heterotopia (ie, the double-cortex syndrome) [Fig. 17].

Another potential area for confusing normal findings for cortical dysplasia is in the perirolandic fissure region. On coronal images, there is often poorer visualization of the gray matter thickness in the perirolandic fissure region compared with the rest of the frontal lobes as well as poor distinction between gray and white matter (Bronen RA, unpublished data). This variation appears to be caused by a combination of factors, one of which is that the

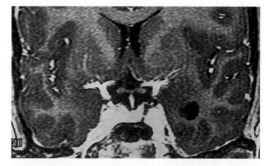

Fig. 15. Uncal recess. The hypointense finding in the left temporal lobe on this contrast-enhanced T1-weighted coronal image could easily be misinterpreted as a cystic lesion. However, it represents CSF in the uncal recess or anterior recess of the temporal horn and is contiguous with the temporal horn (although the bridging CSF may be small). The uncal recess is normally asymmetric in 60% of individuals.

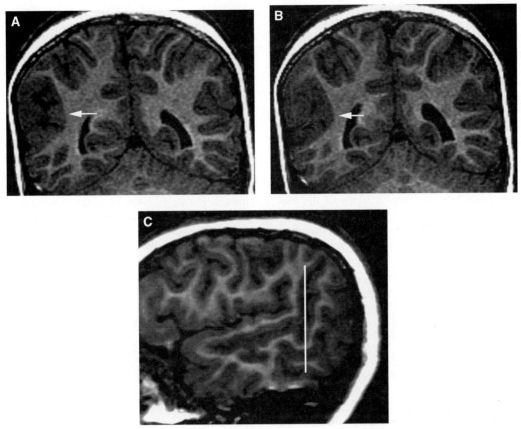

Fig. 16. Polymicrogyria differential diagnosis. Coronal T1-weighted images demonstrate a conglomeration of gray matter (*arrows*) in (*A*) and (*B*), which could represent polymicrogyria. Sagittal reformatted images (*C*) show that this is caused by gray matter along a prominent vertical portion of the posterior extent of the superior temporal sulcus (*line*). The cortical thickness is normal on sagittal images.

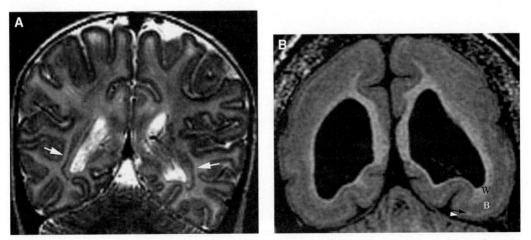

Fig. 17. Band heterotopia differential diagnosis. (*A*) Coronal T2-weighted image shows a bilateral structure (*arrows*) that is isointense to gray matter. This represents myelinated optic radiations against a backdrop of unmyelinated white matter in this infant and should not be confused with band heterotopia. (*B*) Compare with true band heterotopia in (*B*). B, band hetertopia; W, periventricular white matter; black arrow, subcortical white matter; white arrowhead, cortex.

gray matter surrounding the rolandic fissure is normally thinner than cortices in the rest of the brain. Another factor is that the frontal sulci and gyri anterior to the rolandic fissure (ie, superior, middle, and inferior frontal gyri) are perpendicular to the coronal plane, allowing for good definition of their cross-sectional surfaces; whereas the rolandic fissure and adjacent gyri are parallel to the coronal plane, allowing for partial volume effects with white matter. Because of the difficulty interpreting this region on coronal images, reference to axial (or axial reformatted) images should be performed, especially as frontal lobe epilepsy is secondary only to temporal lobe epilepsy in terms of the most common regions of partial seizures.

Other potential sources for errors with interpretation include evaluation of the hippocampus. As previously discussed, the key features of hippocampal sclerosis are hippocampal asymmetry and signal hyperintensity on FLAIR imaging. Artificial hippocampal size asymmetry can be created by head rotation because the cross-sectional size of the hippocampus is greatest anteriorly (at its head) and progressively tapers on more posterior sections. Correct interpretation depends on (1) accurate alignment of the patients head in the scanner and (2) taking head rotation into account for determining hippocampal symmetry in those subjects who fail to be properly aligned [Fig. 18]. Caution is also advised when interpreting FLAIR sequence images. The signal intensity of the hippocampi on FLAIR sequences is slightly greater than the cortex in healthy individuals and this has the potential of leading to a false diagnosis of bilateral hippocam-

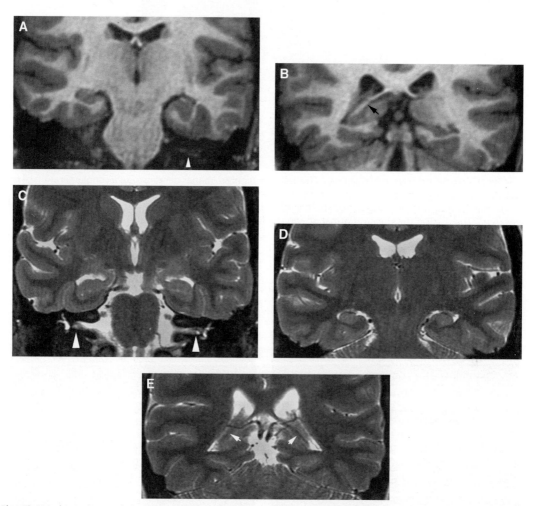

Fig. 18. Head rotation and the hippocampus. On the initial T1-weighted images (*A, B*), the right hippocampus is markedly smaller than the left, suggesting hippocampal sclerosis (*A*). However, this is the result of marked head rotation as confirmed by the marked asymmetry of the internal auditory canal (*arrowhead*) and fornix (*arrow*). After patient repositioning (*C–E*), head rotation is corrected as noted by the symmetry of the IACs (*arrowheads*) and fornices (*arrows*) on the T2-weighted coronal images. With head rotation corrected, there is no longer apparent hippocampal asymmetry.

pal sclerosis in seizure patients. The configuration of the hippocampus can be variable, and this may also lead to difficulties with interpretation. The hippocampal body usually has an oval or round shape in the coronal plane. Infrequently, it may have a more vertical configuration, which may lead to an erroneous diagnosis of cortical dysgenesis. In cases of corpus callosum agenesis or holoprosencephaly, there may be associated incomplete infolding of the cornu ammonis and dentate gyrus, which manifests as a vertically shaped hippocampus with a (shallow) medial cleft on coronal images [Fig. 19].

Differential diagnosis: avoiding the pitfalls

Potential misinterpretations of imaging findings in seizure patients may be due to a number of situations in addition to the normal variations listed above. Perhaps the most troubling are transient lesions, because of the potential for performing lesional resective surgery in a setting where epileptogenesis is either widespread (eg, Rasmussen's encephalitis) or outside the lesional area. Focal transient signal abnormalities in seizure patients may be the result of infections or of prolonged or frequent seizures [20]. Postictal changes can present as focal or multifocal hyperintense abnormalities of the cortex or hippocampus on long TR images and as restricted diffusion (ie, hyperintensity) on diffusion-weighted images [Fig. 20]. Though these latter findings may indicate ischemic changes, perfusion studies show increased blood

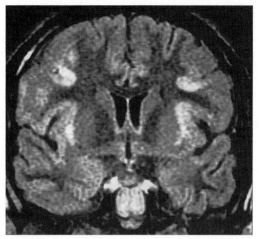

Fig. 20. Postictal changes. Multifocal regions of hyperintensity of the cortex are present on this coronal FLAIR image from a patient that was in status epilepticus. This is more problematic when postictal changes occur in the hippocampus unilaterally.

flow rather than decreased blood flow associated with infarction. In Rasmussen's syndrome, signal changes may not only be transient, but also move from location to location. Therefore, caution should be exercised in interpreting findings and recommending invasive studies for actively seizing patients [21,71]. Morphologic and signal abnormalities are also reported in recurrent focal or febrile seizures in the hippocampus [72,73]. Transient lesions may also affect the splenium of the corpus callosum [74]. This rare isolated focal lesion, occurring in 0.5% epilepsy patients, is characterized by hyperintensity on long TR images, restricted diffusion, and lack of enhancement [Fig. 21]. This par-

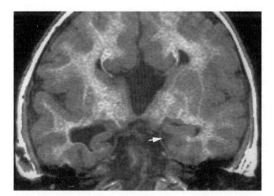

Fig. 19. Unfolded hippocampus. In this patient with agenesis of the corpus callosum, the hippocampi have characteristic features of an unfolded hippocampus—a medial CSF cleft (*arrow*) with a vertically oriented hippocampus, typical of a hippocampus that failed to completely infold the dentate gyrus and cornu ammonis together during development. (*From* Kier EL, Kim JH, Fulbright RK, Bronen RA. Embryology of the human fetal hippocampus: MR imaging, anatomy, and histology. AJNR Am J Neuroradiol 1997;18:525–32; with permission).

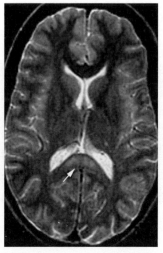

Fig. 21. Splenial signal intensity. Isolated hyperintensity of the splenium of the corpus callosum (*arrow*) on this axial T2-weighted image in this patient with epilepsy.

ticular lesion is thought to result from either frequent seizures or abrupt changes in antiepileptic drug concentrations that may elevate arginine vasopressin and possibly cause cytotoxic edema in the splenium.

Differentiating neoplasms from either focal cortical dysplasia or hippocampal sclerosis may be problematic at times. Hyperintense signal changes on T2-weighted images in the subcortical white matter may be present in neoplasms as well as focal cortical dysplasia (particularly balloon cell focal cortical dysplasia). Surgical strategies may differ for these entities, especially if an epileptogenic lesion is located in an eloquent area of the cortex (ie, primary motor or speech). Imaging findings suggestive of dysplasia rather than neoplasm include cortical thickening, the presence of a radial band extending from lesion to the ventricle, and homogenous appearance of subcortical white matter hyperintensity [see Fig. 3]. High-resolution imaging, perhaps with a high field-strength magnet or phased array surface coils may be helpful for demonstrating cortical thickening. A frontal lobe location is more commonly seen in dysplasias, whereas a temporal lobe location is more commonly seen in tumors. The presence of subependymal or multiple subcortical lesions should raise concerns for tuberous sclerosis.

In individuals with a hyperintense hippocampus on long TR images, practitioners must distinguish tumor from hippocampal sclerosis. This is not particularly difficult if the hippocampus is ipsilaterally small, which represents the cardinal finding of hippocampal sclerosis. However, the hippocampus is not small in all cases of hippocampal sclerosis. Findings suggestive of neoplasm include heterogeneous signal changes and extension of signal changes beyond the hippocampus into the parahippocampal white matter [Fig. 22].

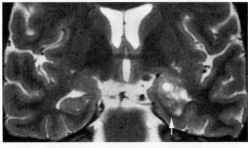

Fig. 22. Hippocampal hyperintensity differential diagnosis. Heterogeneous signal intensity, extension beyond the confines of the hippocampus, and lack of hippocampal atrophy are signs of neoplastic involvement as opposed to hippocampal sclerosis. This heterogeneous hippocampal lesion (*arrow*) was a neoplasm.

Malformations of cortical development can sometimes be difficult to distinguish from one another and from normal structures. Differentiating polymicrogyria from the pachygyria/agyria (lissencephaly) spectrum appears to be a particular problem [compare Figs. 4 and 5]. Both entities present with cortical thickening on imaging, which may be bilateral and appear as smooth cortices (because of the "micro" gyri in polymicrogyria entity). One differentiating feature is the tendency for polymicrogyria to affect the sylvian fissure and to be associated with a CSF cleft. Sagittal images may be particularly helpful—perisylvian polymicrogyria often results in a sylvian fissure that is continuous with the central sulcus, which is easily depicted on the sagittal images. Though polymicrogyria may be bilateral, it is not as diffuse and pervasive as pachygyria (even though pachygyria may affect the brain regionally, such as the frontal lobes). With high-resolution imaging, multiple gyri in polymicrogyria may be visualized.

The differential diagnosis for periventricular findings that are isointense to gray matter on T1-weighted images include periventricular heterotopia, normal caudate nucleus, and subependymal tuberous sclerosis hamartomas. True gray matter follows the signal intensity of the cortex on all pulse sequences, not only T1-weighted sequences. Regarding the caudate nucleus, the head is easily identified, allowing the identification of body and tail on subsequent slices and differentiation from heterotopia.

The asymmetric hemisphere may also be problematic—hemimegalencephaly may sometimes be mistaken for the hemiatrophic syndromes [see Fig. 11]. In both entities, there is ventricular enlargement (and one hemisphere is larger than the other), and there may be diffuse white matter hyperintensity. However, the ventricular enlargement in hemiatrophy is in the smaller hemisphere; ventricular enlargement occurs in the larger hemisphere in hemimegalencephaly. Unlike hemiatrophy, hemimegalencephaly is associated with cortical thickening, sulcal abnormalities, heterotopias, and radial bands.

An important pitfall to avoid relates to dual pathology. As discussed previously, dual pathology refers to the presence of an extrahippocampal lesion and hippocampal sclerosis [Fig. 23]. It is easy to focus on an obvious lesion and neglect assessment of the hippocampus, especially if there are correlative electroclinical features. However, coincidental hippocampal sclerosis is not infrequent, especially with developmental anomalies.

The temporal lobe encephalocele is an extremely rare cause of epilepsy that can lead to errors in interpretation (occurring in 1 of 600 patients who have undergone epilepsy surgery in the last 18 years

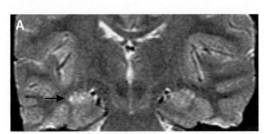
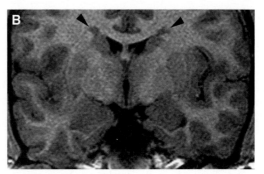

Fig. 23. Dual pathology. (*A*) Coronal T2-weighted image shows findings of hippocampal sclerosis—hippocampal atrophy and hyperintensity (*arrow*). (*B*) Coronal T1-weighted image in this same patient demonstrates an additional finding of bilateral heterotopia (*arrowheads*).

at the authors' institution). Because it occupies an extra-axial location, it is easily overlooked unless the basal temporal lobe is specifically scrutinized for this disorder. The need to distinguish this pathologic condition from the normal protrusions of brain tissue occurring along the basal temporal lobes is important [Fig. 24].

Postoperative imaging

MR imaging plays a crucial role not only in the presurgical evaluation of patients with medically refractory epilepsy but also in the postoperative imaging of these patients. MR imaging can determine the extent of surgical resection for epileptogenic substrates and surgical divisions for functional hemispherectomies. In patients who have not had success with surgery, MR imaging can identify (1) residual substrate at the operative site, (2) any other previously unrecognized epileptogenic substrates at other locations in the brain,

and (3) persistent connections in functional hemispherectomies [11].

Knowledge of the normal patterns of enhancement is essential to avoid misinterpretation of the benign findings in the postoperative MR imaging scans. During the first postoperative week, a thin linear enhancement can be seen at the pial margins of the resection site [75]. In those with temporal lobe surgery, enlargement and enhancement of the choroid plexus occurs on the ipsilateral side [76]. Pneumocephalus is commonly present during the first 4 to 5 days after surgery. In patients with persistence of this finding after 5 days, a fistula or infectious process may need to be excluded.

One week to 1 month after surgery, the resection margin enhances with a thick linear or nodular pattern and may mimic residual neoplastic or inflammatory processes [Fig. 25]. Sometime between 1 month and 3 to 5 months after surgery, the

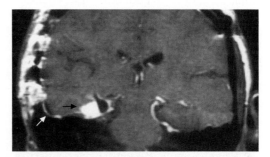

Fig. 25. Postoperative enhancement. Coronal enhanced image 3 weeks after temporal lobectomy for hippocampal sclerosis shows nodular enhancement (*black arrow*) that could be mistaken for tumor, if this resection had been performed for a neoplasm. Dural enhancement (*white arrow*) is usually seen postoperatively as well. (*From* Sato N, Bronen RA, Sze G, Kawamura Y, Coughlin W, Putman CM, et al. Postoperative changes in the brain: MR imaging findings in patients without neoplasms. Radiology 1997;204(3): 839–46; with permission.)

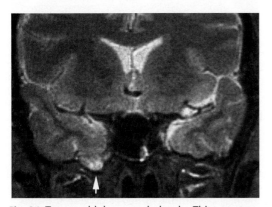

Fig. 24. Temporal lobe encephalocele. This rare cause of temporal lobe epilepsy was visualized retrospectively on MR (*arrow*) after it was discovered at surgery. This is easily overlooked when concentrating on the hippocampus and cortex, if it is not scrutinized for prospectively.

resection margin stops enhancing. The course for dural enhancement mimics that of pial enhancement, except that dural enhancement persists and can last for years [75].

MR imaging is more sensitive in detecting complications of hemispherectomy, such as extra- or intra-axial hemorrhage, hydrocephalus, or infections. MR imaging can also demonstrate sequela of placement of intraparenchymal depth electrodes. Punctate hyperintense signal abnormalities on long TR sequences can be seen in these cases, representing gliosis along the tracks of the electrode [77]. Rarely, punctate hemosiderin is visualized along a depth electrode tract, representing evidence of prior hemorrhage.

Interpretation of MR images: a systematic approach

Many epileptogenic lesions are subtle and can be easily missed unless a systematic approach is used during the interpretation of MR images from a seizure patient [43]. One approach can be followed using the mnemonic "HIPPO SAGE" [Box 2]. The hypothalamus is reviewed to detect a hypothalamic hamartomas, particularly in children. These can be subtle and overlooked, especially if the patient does not present with gelastic seizures [Fig. 26]. Hippocampal size, symmetry, and signal abnormalities are assessed in the coronal plane to evaluate for hippocampal sclerosis. Because head rotation may lead to a false diagnosis of hippocampal atrophy, head rotation is assessed based on symmetry of the internal auditory canals and symmetry of the atria of the left lateral ventricles [see Fig. 18]. If head rotation is present, assessment of hippocampal symmetry must be compensated for by comparing compatible coronal hippocampal sections (ie, the right hippocampal section adjacent to the right internal auditory canal should be compared with left hippocampal section adjacent to the left internal auditory canal). Periventricular regions should be scrutinized for subependymal gray matter het-

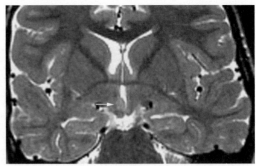

Fig. 26. Hypothalamic hamartoma. Coronal T2-weighted image shows a hypothalamic hamartoma (*white arrow*), causing mass effect on the third ventricle and ipsilateral mammillary body. This patient presented with right frontal seizures, and this lesion was not detected on the initial MR study because the hypothalamus was not scrutinized. It was detected on this subsequent MR study after the seizures took on a gelastic quality.

erotopias, which occur most commonly adjacent to the atria of lateral ventricles. Gray matter inferiorlateral to the temporal horns is abnormal [see Fig. 4; Fig. 27].

Because focal epilepsy is a cortical-based process, the periphery of the brain should be carefully scrutinized for developmental anomalies, atrophic processes, and small neoplasms or vascular malformations. The authors closely inspect for the sulcal and gyral morphologic changes (which underlie developmental disorders) [Fig. 28], atrophic processes (which may underlie glottic substrates or represent developmental CSF clefts) [see Fig. 8], and gray matter thickening and indistinctness of

---

Box 2: Systematic evaluation of MR scans of seizure patients (HIPPO SAGE)

- Hypothalamic hamartoma; hippocampal size and signal abnormality
- Internal auditory canal and atrial assymmetry
- Periventricular heterotopia
- Peripheral abnormalities
  - Sulcal morphologic abnormalities
  - Atrophy
  - Gray matter thickening
  - Encephalocele of anterior temporal lobe
- Obvious lesion

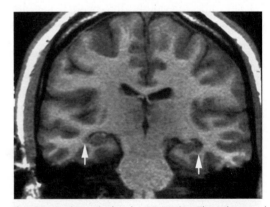

Fig. 27. Periventricular heterotopia. The abnormal gray matter (*arrows*) on this coronal T1-weighted image may be difficult to detect because it blends in with the normal gray matter of the hippocampus. The periventricular regions need to be scrutinized for heterotopia in all seizure patients. (*From* Bronen RA, Fulbright RK, Kim JH, et al. A systematic approach for interpreting MR images of the seizure patient. AJR Am J Roentgenol 1997;169(1):241–7; with permission).

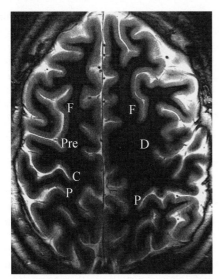

Fig. 28. Sulcal morphologic changes, cortical dysplasia. The perirolandic region is a common location for frontal lobe dysplasias causing epilepsy. Detection requires assessment of the normal cortical anatomy on axial images. This inversion recovery image shows the normal perirolandic fissure configurations on the right side, the superior frontal sulcus (F), precentral sulcus (Pre), central sulcus (C), and postcentral sulcus (P). On the left side, the normal anatomic configuration is distorted by the dysplastic cortex (D), which has caused loss of the typical superior frontal, precentral, and central sulci pattern.

gray-white matter junction (associated with developmental disorders) [see Figs. 3–5, 11C]. The inferior aspect of the anterior temporal lobe is assessed to exclude a temporal lobe encephalocele, an extremely uncommon cause of epilepsy but one that is easily overlooked if not specifically assessed for [see Fig. 24] [43].

Finally, the authors evaluate the obvious lesion in the brain and assess its characteristics. The obvious lesion could be an incidental finding, an epileptogenic substrate, or an additional lesion. By concen-

trating only on an obvious lesion, there is a chance that concurring hippocampal sclerosis will not be detected in those patients with dual pathology [see Figs. 2 and 23].

Recommendations for imaging protocols

Most standard or routine MR imaging protocols typically used to evaluate intracranial disease are suboptimal in the identification of epileptogenic substrates, such as cortical dysplasia, hippocampal sclerosis, and band heterotopia [78]. Optimal imaging parameters (image orientation, slice thickness, and pulse sequences) need to be employed to identify these substrates [Fig. 29].

With regard to hippocampal sclerosis, the most ideal plane for depicting the findings of hippocampal atrophy, signal changes and disruption of internal architecture is the oblique coronal (ie, the imaging plane perpendicular to the long axis of the hippocampus). FLAIR sequences appear to have the best sensitivity for demonstrating abnormal signal in the hippocampus [79], though the authors use a combination of coronal FLAIR and fast spin echo T2-weighted sequences to assess signal intensity because the hippocampus is normally slightly hyper-intense compared with gray matter on FLAIR sequences in certain individuals [80], making interpretation difficult if relying solely on the FLAIR images. Most epileptic centers employ T1-weighted gradient volume acquisitions (SPGR or MP-RAGE) to help assess the morphology of the hippocampus and to evaluate for developmental disorders. The raw data from these high-resolution images can be reconstructed in any plane and aid in qualitative, morphometric, and volumetric analysis of the hippocampus. Inversion recovery sequences with good gray/white matter differentiation also provide information regarding morphology and signal abnormalities. Some centers use T2 relaxometry or spectroscopy to further assess the hippocampus and medial temporal lobes. T2 relaxometry

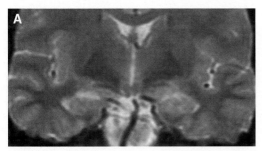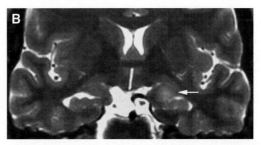

Fig. 29. Technique. Coronal T2-weighted images demonstrate the value of high-quality techniques for detecting epileptogenic abnormalities. (A) The left temporal lobe lesion cannot be visualized on this 5-mm thick slice with a gap of 2.5 mm (ie, effective slice thickness of 7.5 mm) and a 256 × 192 matrix. (B) On this higher resolution image, the lesion (arrow) is easily seen on this and adjacent sections. This scan was performed with 3-mm thick contiguous slices and a 256 × 256 matrix.

is useful in cases where the findings on visual analysis are equivocal or in lateralization of seizure focus when bilateral abnormalities exist in the hippocampi.

Recommended sequences for developmental anomalies include FLAIR sequence to assess for hyperintense signal changes and radial bands and a sequence capable of depicting good contrast between gray matter and white matter, particularly with thin slices. Malformations of cortical development are subtle abnormalities and can be missed easily without employing high-resolution imaging and sequences with good gray/white matter differentiation [81,82]. Coronal T1-weighted gradient volume sequences (SPGR or MP-RAGE) with thin slice thickness (1 to 1.6 mm) can demonstrate subtle developmental malformations [83]. There are many additional measures that can be used to increase the yield for detecting MCD. Postprocessing of the raw data from a 3D volume set can yield high-resolution 3D reformations, which can demonstrate cortical dysplasia, abnormal sulcal morphology, gray/white matter indistinctiveness, and the relationship of developmental abnormalities to the eloquent cortical regions [84]. High-resolution imaging with phased array coils, image registration and averaging, and high-field scanners (greater than 3T) can provide adequate information in locating the cortical dysplasia [81,82]. FLAIR/T2-weighted images demonstrate abnormal signal in the subcortical/deep white matter associated with developmental malformations. Quantitative analysis of gray and white matter, when compared with normal controls, may show widespread developmental abnormalities. However, the location and extent of cortical dysplasia identified by MR imaging may not correlate with the seizure semiology or the electrophysiologic studies [34].

Routine use of intravenous contrast (gadolinium) is not indicated in the evaluation of chronic epilepsy patients but may play a role in the evaluation of patients with new onset of epilepsy to look for infectious, inflammatory and neoplastic processes, especially in those over 50 years old [85–87]. One clear exception to this is in the patient with hemiatrophy, where contrast may diagnose Sturge-Weber syndrome [see **Fig. 11**]. However, after identification of a lesion on MR imaging, contrast is often helpful. Infusion of intravenous contrast increases the diagnostic confidence, delineates the extent of lesion, differentiates between an aggressive and a nonaggressive lesion, and may be useful for guidance for obtaining the biopsy specimen [86].

Some techniques appear to be useful, but are not easily implemented on a routine basis or early in the evaluation process. Apparent diffusion coefficient maps and diffusion tensor imaging can identify the abnormal diffusion at the epileptogenic foci in normal-appearing standard MR imaging studies [88–90]. Abnormal magnetization transfer ratios in epilepsy patients with negative conventional MR imaging may detect and delineate the extent of occult malformations of cortical development [91]. Various image analysis, segmentation, and quantitative techniques have shown benefits in the detection of epileptogenic abnormalities but are not routinely available with commercial clinical MR scanners or work stations. Functional MR imaging is useful in preoperative localization of the motor strip in relation to the epileptogenic foci in this region [92]. fMR imaging information of lateralization of memory and language is promising and may be useful in the prediction of postsurgical seizure relief and cognitive deficits after anterior temporal lobectomy [93]. fMR imaging has also been shown to detect the cortical activation in the brain before the clinical seizure activity, but this appears to be a rare finding [94].

Summary

MR imaging plays a pivotal role in the evaluation of patients with epilepsy. With its high spatial resolution, excellent inherent soft tissue contrast, multiplanar imaging capability, and lack of ionizing radiation, MR imaging has emerged as a versatile diagnostic tool in the evaluation of patients with epilepsy. MR imaging not only identifies specific epileptogenic substrates but also determines specific treatment and predicts prognosis. Employing appropriate imaging protocols and reviewing the images in a systematic manner helps in the identification of subtle epileptogenic structural abnormalities. With future improvements in software, hardware, and post-processing methods, MR imaging should be able to throw more light on epileptogenesis and help physicians to better understand its structural basis.

References

[1] Commission on Classification and Terminology of the International League against Epilepsy. Proposal for revised classification of epilepsies and epileptic syndromes. Epilepsia 1989;30:389–99.

[2] Kwan P, Brodie M. Early identification of refractory epilepsy. N Engl J Med 2000;342:314–9.

[3] Arroyo S. Evaluation of drug-resistant epilepsy. Rev Neurol 2000;30:881–9.

[4] Bell GS, Sander JW. The epidemiology of epilepsy: the size of the problem. Seizure 2001;16:165–70.

[5] Sander JW. The epidemiology of epilepsy revisited. Curr Opin Neurol 2003;16:165–70.

[6] Bernal B, Altman N. Evidence-based medicine: neuroimaging of seizures. Neuroimaging Clin N Am 2003;13:211–24.

[7] King MA, Newton MR, Jackson GD, et al. Epileptology of the first-seizure presentation: a clinical, electroencephalographic, and magnetic resonance imaging study of 300 consecutive patients [see comment]. Lancet 1998;352:1007–11.

[8] Berg A, Testa FM, Levy SR. Neuroimaging in children with newly diagnosed epilepsy: a community based study. Pediatrics 2000;106:527–32.

[9] Bronen RA, Fulbright RK, Spencer DD, et al. Refractory epilepsy: comparison of MR imaging, CT, and histopathologic findings in 117 patients. Radiology 1996;201:97–105.

[10] Scott CA, Fish DR, Smith SJ, et al. Presurgical evaluation of patients with epilepsy and normal MRI: role of scalp video-EEG telemetry [see comment]. J Neurol Neurosurg Psychiatry 1999;66:69–71.

[11] Commission on Neuroimaging of the International League against Epilepsy. Guidelines for neuroimaging evaluation of patients with uncontrolled epilepsy considered for surgery. Epilepsia 1998;39:1375–6.

[12] Commission on Neuroimaging of the International League against Epilepsy. Recommendations for neuroimaging of patients with epilepsy. Epilepsia 1997;38:1255–6.

[13] Anonymous. Practice parameter: the neurodiagnostic evaluation of the child with a first simple febrile seizure. Pediatrics 1996;97:769–75.

[14] Anonymous. Practice parameter: neuroimaging in the emergency patient presenting with seizure. Summary statement. Neurology 1996;47:288–91.

[15] Holmes MD, Wilensky AJ, Ojemann GA, Ojemann LM. Hippocampal or neocortical lesions on magnetic resonance imaging do not necessarily indicate site of ictal onsets in partial epilepsy. Ann Neurol 1999;45:461–5.

[16] Berkovic SF, McIntosh AM, Kalnios RM, et al. Preoperative MRI predicts outcome of temporal lobectomy: an actuarial analysis. Neurology 1995;45:1358–63.

[17] Spencer D. Classifying the epilepsies by substrate. Clin Neurosci 1994;2:104–9.

[18] Spencer SS. When should temporal lobe epilepsy be treated surgically? Lancet Neurol 2002;1:375–82.

[19] Jackson G, VanPaesschen W. Hippocampal sclerosis in the MR era. Epilepsia 2002;43:4–10.

[20] Bronen RA. Epilepsy: the role of MR imaging. AJR Am J Roentgenol 1992;159:1165–74.

[21] Bronen RA, Gupta V. Epilepsy. In: Atlas S, editor. MRI of brain and spine. New York: Lippincott Williams & Wilkins; 2002. p. 415–55.

[22] Jack CJ, Sharbrough FW, Cascino GD, et al. Magnetic resonance image-based hippocampal volumetry: correlation with outcome after temporal lobectomy. Ann Neurol 1992;31:138–46.

[23] Oppenheim C, Dormont D, Biondi A, et al. Loss of digitations of the hippocampal head on high resolution fast spin echo MR: a sign of mesial temporal sclerosis. AJNR Am J Neuroradiol 1998;19:457–63.

[24] Baldwin GN, Tsuruda JS, Maravilla KR, et al. The fornix in patients with seizures caused by unilateral hippocampal sclerosis: detection of unilateral volume loss on MR images. AJR Am J Roentgenol 1994;162:1185–9.

[25] Meiners LC, Witkamp TD, de Kort GA, et al. Relevance of temporal lobe white matter changes in hippocampal sclerosis. Magnetic resonance imaging and histology. Invest Radiol 1999;34:38–45.

[26] Jack CJ, Sharbrough FW, Twomey CK, et al. Temporal lobe seizures: lateralization with MR volume measurements of the hippocampal formation. Radiology 1990;175:423–9.

[27] Bronen RA, Anderson AW, Spencer DD. Quantitative MR for epilepsy: a clinical and research tool? AJNR Am J Neuroradiol 1994;15:1157–60.

[28] Jack Jr CR. MRI-based hippocampal volume measurements in epilepsy. Epilepsia 1994;35:S21–9.

[29] Arruda F, Cendes F, Andermann F, et al. Mesial atrophy and outcome after amygdalohippocampectomy or temporal lobe removal. Ann Neurol 1996;40:446–50.

[30] Quigg M, Bertram EH, Jackson T, Laws E. Volumetric magnetic resonance imaging evidence of bilateral hippocampal atrophy in mesial temporal lobe epilepsy. Epilepsia 1997;38:588–94.

[31] Cendes F, Cook MJ, Watson C, et al. Frequency and characteristics of dual pathology in patients with lesional epilepsy. Neurology 1995;45:2058–64.

[32] Sisodiya SM, Moran N, Free SL, et al. Correlation of widespread pre-operative magnetic resonance imaging changes with unsuccessful surgery for hippocampal sclerosis. Ann Neurol 1997;41:490–6.

[33] Li LM, Cendes F, Andermann F, et al. Surgical outcome in patients with epilepsy and dual pathology. Brain 1999;122:799–805.

[34] Raymond AA, Fish DR, Sisodiya SM, et al. Abnormalities of gyration, heterotopias, tuberous sclerosis, focal cortical dysplasia, microdysgenesis, dysembryo-plastic neuroepithelial tumour and dysgenesis of the archicortex in epilepsy. Clinical, EEG and neuroimaging features in 100 adult patients. Brain 1995;118:629–60.

[35] Kuzniecky R. Magnetic resonance imaging in cerebral developmental malformations and epilepsy. In: Cascino GD, Jack CJ, editors. Neuroimaging in epilepsy: principles and practice. Newton (MA): Butterworth-Heinemann; 1996. p. 51–63.

[36] Wyllie E, Comair YG, Kotagal P. Seizure outcome after epilepsy surgery in children and adolescents. Ann Neurol 1998;44:740–8.

[37] Barkovich AJ, Kuzniecky RI, Jackson GD, et al. Classification system for malformation of cortical development: update 2001. Neurology 2001;57:2168–78.

[38] Barkovich AJ. Congenital malformations of the brain and skull. In: Barkovich A, editor. Pediatric imaging. New York: Lippincott Williams & Wilkins; 2000. p. 251–381.

[39] Bronen RA, Spencer DD, Fulbright RK. Cerebrospinal fluid cleft with cortical dimple: MR imaging marker for focal cortical dysgenesis. Radiology 2000;214:657–63.

[40] Palmini A, Gambardella A, Andermann F, et al. Operative strategies for patients with cortical dysplastic lesions and intractable epilepsy. Epilepsia 1994;35:S57–71.

[41] Sisodiya SM, Free SL, Stevens JM, et al. Widespread cerebral structural changes in patients with cortical dysgenesis and epilepsy. Brain 1995; 118:1039–50.

[42] Cascino G. Selection of candidates for surgical treatment of epilepsy. In: Cascino G, Jack CJ, editors. Neuroimaging in epilepsy: principles and practice. Newton (MA): Butterworth-Heinemann; 1996. p. 219–34.

[43] Bronen RA, Fulbright RK, Kim JH, et al. A systematic approach for interpreting MR images of the seizure patient. AJR Am J Roentgenol 1997;169:241–7.

[44] Bronen RA, Fulbright RK, Spencer DD, et al. MR characteristics of neoplasms and vascular malformations associated with epilepsy. Magn Reson Imaging 1995;13:1153–62.

[45] Friedland R, Bronen R. Magnetic resonance imaging of neoplastic, vascular, and indeterminate substrates. In: Cascino G, Jack CJ, editors. Neuroimaging in epilepsy: principles and practice. Newton (MA): Butterworth-Heinemann; 1996. p. 29–50.

[46] Atlas S, Lavi E, Fisher P. Intra-axial brain tumors. In: Atlas S, editor. MRI of the brain and spine. New York: Lippincott Williams & Wilkins; 2002. p. 565–693.

[47] Koeller KK, Henry JM. From the archives of the AFIP Superficial gliomas: radiologic-pathologic correlation. Radiographics 2001;21:1533–56.

[48] Provanzale J. Comparison of patient age with MR imaging features of gangliogliomas. AJR Am J Roentgenol 2000;174:859–62.

[49] Piepgras DG, Sundt TJ, Ragoowansi AT, Stevens L. Seizure outcome in patients with surgically treated cerebral arteriovenous malformations. J Neurosurg 1993;78:5–11.

[50] Rivera PP, Willinsky RA. Intracranial cavernous malformations. Neuroimaging Clin N Am 2003; 13:27–40.

[51] Bladin CF, Alexandrov AV, Bellavance A, et al, for the Seizures after Stroke Study Group. Seizures after stroke. Arch Neurol 2000;57:1617–22.

[52] Ho SS, Kuzniecky RI. Congenital porencephaly: MR features and relationship to hippocampal sclerosis. AJNR Am J Neuroradiol 1998;19:135–41.

[53] Barkovich AJ. Brain and spine injuries in infancy and childhood. In: Barkovich A, editor. Pediatric neuroimaging. New York: Lippincott Williams & Wilkins; 2000. p. 157–249.

[54] Kuzniecky R, Jackson G. Disorders of cerebral hemispheres. In: Kuzniecky R, Jackson G, editors. Magnetic resonance in epilepsy. New York: Raven-Press; 1995. p. 213–33.

[55] Annegers J. A population based study of seizures after traumatic brain injuries. N Engl J Med 1998; 338:20–4.

[56] Hardman JM, Manoukian A. Pathology of head trauma. Neuroimaging Clin N Am 2002;12: 175–87.

[57] Willmore LJ. Post-traumatic epilepsy: cellular mechanisms and implications for treatment. Epilepsia 1990;31:s67–73.

[58] Frey LC. Epidemiology of posttraumatic epilepsy: a critical review. Epilepsia 2003;44(Suppl 10): 11–7.

[59] White Jr AC. Neurocysticercosis: updates on epidemiolgy, pathogenesis, diagnosis, and management. Annu Rev Med 2000;51:187–206.

[60] Shah G. Central nervous system tuberculosis: imaging manifestations. Neuroimaging Clin N Am 2000;10:355–74.

[61] Bien CG, Widman G, Urbach H, et al. The natural history of Rasmussen's encephalitis. Brain 2002;125:1751–9.

[62] Chiapparini L, Granata T, Farina L, et al. Diagnostic imaging in 13 cases of Rasmussen's encephalitis: can early MRI suggest the diagnosis? Neuroradiology 2003;45:171–83.

[63] Barkovich AJ. The phakomatoses. In: Barkovich AJ, editor. Pediatric neuroimaging. New York: Lippincott Williams & Wilkins; 2000. p. 383–441.

[64] Arroyo S, Santamaria J. What is the relationship between arachnoid cysts and seizure foci? [see comment]. Epilepsia 1997;38:1098–102.

[65] Song CJ, Kim JH, Kier EL, Bronen RA. MR imaging and histologic features of subinsular bright spots on T2-weighted MR images: Virchow-Robin spaces of the extreme capsule and insular cortex. Radiology 2000;214:671–7.

[66] Kier EL, Kim JH, Fulbright RK, Bronen RA. Embryology of the human fetal hippocampus: MR imaging, anatomy, and histology. AJNR Am J Neuroradiol 1997;18:525–32.

[67] Sasaki M, Sone M, Ehara S, Tamakawa Y. Hippocampal sulcus remnant: potential cause of change in signal intensity in the hippocampus. Radiology 1993;188:743–6.

[68] Topper R, Jurgens E, Reul J, Thron A. Clinical significance of intracranial developmental venous anomalies. J Neurol Neurosurg Psychiatry 1999;67:234–8.

[69] Naff NJ, Wemmer J, Hoenig-Rigamonti DR. A longitudinal study of patients with venous malformations: documentation of a negligible hemorrhage risk and benign natural history. Neurology 1998;50:1709–14.

[70] Savas R, Sener RN. Deep calcarine sulcus and prominent calcar avis. J Neuroradiol 1998;25: 144–6.

[71] Chan S, Chin SS, Kartha K, et al. Reversible signal abnormalities in the hippocampus and neocor-

tex after prolonged seizures. AJNR Am J Neuroradiol 1996;17:1725–31.

[72] Tien RD, Felsberg GJ. The hippocampus in status epilepticus; demonstration of signal intensity and morphologic changes with sequential fast spin-echo MR imaging. Radiology 1995;194:249–56.

[73] VanLandingham KE, Heinz ER, Cavazos JE, et al. Magnetic resonance imaging evidence of hippocampal injury after prolonged focal febrile convulsions. Ann Neurol 1998;43:413–26.

[74] Mirsattari SM, Lee DH, Jones MW, et al. Transient lesion in the splenium of the corpus collosum in an epileptic patient. Neurology 2003;60:1838–41.

[75] Sato N, Bronen RA, Sze G, et al. Postoperative changes in the brain: MR imaging findings in patients without neoplasms. Radiology 1997;204:839–46.

[76] Saluja S, Sato N, Kawamura Y, et al. Choroid plexus changes after temporal lobectomy. AJNR Am J Neuroradiol 2000;21:1650–3.

[77] Merriam MA, Bronen RA, Spencer DD, McCarthy G. MR findings after depth electrode implantation for medically refractory epilepsy. AJNR Am J Neuroradiol 1993;14:1343–6.

[78] McBride MC, Bronstein KS, Bennett B, et al. Failure of standard magnetic resonance imaging in patients with refractory temporal lobe epilepsy. Arch Neurol 1998;55:346–8.

[79] Jack Jr CR, Rydberg CH, Krecke KN, et al. Mesial temporal sclerosis: diagnosis with fluid-attenuated in-version-recovery versus spin-echo MR imaging. Radiology 1996;199:367–73.

[80] Hirai T, Yoshizunmi K, Shigematsu Y, et al. Limbic lobe of the human brain: evaluation with turbo fluid inversion-recovery MR imaging. Radiology 2000;215:470–5.

[81] Bronen RA, Knowlton R, Garwood M, et al. High resolution imaging in epilepsy. Epilepsia 2002;43:11–8.

[82] Grant PE, Barkovich AJ, Wald LL, et al. High-resolution surface-coil MR of cortical lesions in medically refractory epilepsy: a prospective study. AJNR Am J Neuroradiol 1997;18:291–301.

[83] Barkovich AJ, Rowley HA, Andermann F. MR in partial epilepsy: value of high resolution volumetric techniques. AJNR Am J Neuroradiol 1995;16:339–44.

[84] Ruggieri PM, Najm I, Bronen R, Campos M, Cendes F, Duncan JS, et al. Neuroimaging of the cortical dysplasias. Neurology 2004;62(6 Suppl 3):S27–9.

[85] Bronen RA. Is there any role for gadopentetate dime-glumine administration when searching for mesial temporal sclerosis in patients with seizures? AJR Am J Roentgenol 1995;164:503.

[86] Bradley WG, Shey RB. MR imaging evaluation of seizures. Radiology 2000;214:651–6.

[87] Elster AD, Mirza W. MR imaging in chronic partial epilepsy: role of contrast enhancement. AJNR Am J Neuroradiol 1991;12:165–70.

[88] Rugg-Gunn FJ, Eriksson SH, Symms MR, et al. Diffusion tensor imaging in refractory epilepsy. Lancet 2002;359:1748–51.

[89] Yoo SY CK, Song IC, Han MH, et al. Apparent diffusion coefficient value of the hippocampus in patients with hippocampal sclerosis and in healthy volunteers. AJNR Am J Neuroradiol 2002;23:809–12.

[90] Wieshmann UC, Clark CA, Symms MR, et al. Water diffusion in the human hippocampus in epilepsy. Magn Reson Imaging 1999;17:29–36.

[91] Rugg-Gunn FJ, Eriksson SH, Symms MR, et al. Magnetization transfer imaging in focal epilepsy. Neurology 2003;60:1638–45.

[92] Hollaway V, Chong WK, Connelly A. Somatomotor fMRI in the presurgical evaluation of a case of focal epilepsy. Clin Radiol 1999;54:301–3.

[93] Killgore WD, Glosser G, Casasanto DJ, et al. Functional MRI and the Wada test provide complementary information for predicting postoperative seizure control. Seizure 1999;8:450–5.

[94] Jackson GD, Connelly A, Cross JH, et al. Functional magnetic resonance imaging of focal seizures. Neurology 1994;44:850–6.

RADIOLOGIC
CLINICS
OF NORTH AMERICA

Radiol Clin N Am 44 (2006) 135–157

Anatomy and Pathology of the Eye: Role of MR Imaging and CT

Mahmood F. Mafee, MD[a],*, Afshin Karimi, MD, PhD, JD[b],
Jay Shah, BS[b], Mark Rapoport, BS[b], Sameer A. Ansari, MD, PhD[b]

Since the development of CT and MR imaging, significant progress has been made in ophthalmic imaging. As the technology advanced and MR imaging units improved their ability in terms of spatial resolution, the role of MR imaging in ophthalmic imaging has increased accordingly. This article considers the role of MR and CT imaging in the diagnosis of selected pathologies of the eye.

Ocular anatomy

The globe is formed from the neuroectoderm of the forebrain (prosencephalon), the surface ectoderm of the head, the mesoderm lying between these layers,

and neural crest cells [1–4]. The neuroectoderm gives rise to the retina, the fibers of the optic nerve, and smooth muscles (the sphincter and dilator papillae) of the iris [3]. The surface ectoderm on the side of the head forms the corneal and conjunctival epithelium, the lens, and the lacrimal and tarsal glands [1–4]. The surrounding mesenchyme forms the corneal stroma, the sclera, the choroids, the iris, the ciliary musculature, part of the vitreous body, and the cells lining the anterior chamber [1,4]. The eyeball (eye, globe) is made up of three primary layers [Fig. 1]: (1) the sclera, or outer layer, which is composed of collagen-elastic tissue; (2) the uvea (uveal tract), or middle layer, which is richly vascu-

This article was originally published in *Neuroimaging Clinics of North America* 15:23–47, 2005.
[a] Department of Radiology, University of Illinois at Chicago Medical Center, Chicago, IL, USA
[b] Department of Radiology, University of Illinois Hospital at Chicago, University of Illinois College of Medicine, Chicago, IL, USA
* Corresponding author. Department of Radiology, University of Illinois at Chicago Medical Center, 1740 West Taylor Street, MC 931, Chicago, IL 60612.
E-mail address: mfmafee@uic.edu (M.F. Mafee).

doi:10.1016/j.rcl.2005.09.001

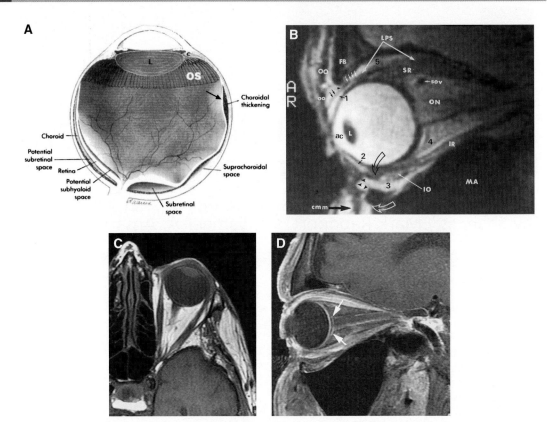

Fig. 1. (*A*) Ocular structures and various intraocular potential spaces. C, ciliary body; L, lens; OS, ora serrata. (*Modified from* Mafee MF, Inoue Y, Mafee RF. Ocular and orbital imaging. Neuroimaging Clin North Am 1996;6:292.) (*B*) Sagittal T2-weighted MR image (1.5 T) shows fibers of orbicilaris oculi (OO), frontal bone (FB), levator palpebrae superioris (LPS), extraconal fat (5), superior rectus muscle (SR), superior ophthalmic vein (SOV), optic nerve (ON), intraconal fatty reticulum (4), inferior rectus muscle (IR), maxillary antrum (MA), inferior oblique muscle (IO), extraconal fat (3), anterior wall of maxillary sinus (*white open arrow*), complex muscles of the mouth (cmm), orbital septum (*arrowheads*), presumed suspensory ligament of Lockwood (*black open arrow*), inferior (2) and superior fornices (1), anterior chamber (ac), lens (L), superior tarsal plate (*black arrows*), and the tendon of insertion of levator palpebrae superioris (*white arrows*). This tendon is an aponeurosis that descends posterior to the orbital septum (the orbital septum is depicted as an ill-defined image [*arrowhead*] in this section). The tendinous fibers then pierce the orbital septum and become attached to the anterior surface of the superior tarsal plate. Some of its fibers pass forward between the muscle bundles of the orbicularis oculi (OO) to attach to the skin. (*From* Mafee MF, Valvassori GE, Becker M, editors. Imaging of the head and neck. Stuttgart (Germany): Thieme; 2005; with permission.) (*C*) Axial T1-weighted image (566/12 ms, repetition time/echo time [TR/TE], 2.5-mm thick section, 352 × 192 matrix, 2 NEX, 160 × 160–mm field of view) obtained on a 3-T MR imaging unit, using eight-channel head coil, showing normal eye and orbit. (*D*) Sagittal fat-suppressed T1-weighted image (416/12 ms, TR/TE, 3-mm thick section, 320 × 192 matrix, 2 NEX, 140 × 140–mm field of view) obtained on a 3-T MR imaging unit using eight-channel head coil, showing normal eye and orbit. Note normal enhancement of uveoretinal coat and optic nerve meninges. Arrows point most likely to chemical shift artifact, rather than Tenon's capsule enhancement.

lar and contains pigmented tissue consisting of the choroid, ciliary body, and iris; and (3) the retina, or inner layer, which is the neural, sensory stratum of the eye. The eyeball is enveloped by a fascial sheath, known as the "fascia bulbi" or "Tenon's capsule." Tenon's capsule forms a socket for the eyeball and is separated from the sclera by Tenon's (episcleral) space [5]. Tenon's capsule is perforated near the equator by the vortex (vorticose) veins, the draining veins of the choroid and sclera [1,5]. Tenon's capsule is also perforated by the optic nerve and its sheath,

the ciliary nerves and vessels. Tenon's capsule fuses with the sclera and the sheath of the optic nerve around the entrance of the optic nerve [5]. Tenon's capsule blends with the sclera just behind the corneoscleral junction and fuses with the bulbar conjunctiva [1]. The tendons of the extrinsic ocular muscles pierce Tenon's capsule to reach the sclera. At the site of perforation, Tenon's capsule is reflected back along these muscle sheaths to form a tubular sleeve [6]. The connection between the muscle fibers, sheath, and the tubular sheath is especially strong at the point where the two fuse [5,6]. For this reason, the muscles retain their attachment to the capsule and do not retract extensively after enucleation (tenotomy) [5,6].

Sclera

The sclera is the outer supporting layer of the globe, extending from the limbus at the margin of the cornea to the optic nerve, where it becomes continuous with the dural sheath of the optic nerve [1]. The potential episcleral (Tenon's) space is between the outer aspect of the sclera and inner aspect of Tenon's capsule. The potential suprachoroidal space is between the inner aspect of the sclera and the outer aspect of the choroid [1,2]. In adults the sclera is 1 mm thick posteriorly, thinning at the equator to 0.6 mm. It is thinnest (0.3 mm) immediately posterior to the tendinous insertions of the rectus muscles [1,2]. The posterior scleral foramen is the site of scleral perforation by the optic nerve. At this site, the sclera is fused with the dural and arachnoid sheaths of the optic nerve. The lamina cribrosa is where the optic nerve fibers pierce the sclera.

Uvea (choroid, ciliary body, and iris)

The uveal tract (from the Latin *uva* or grape) is a pigmented vascular layer that lies between the sclera and the retina [see Fig. 1]. It consists of the choroid, the ciliary body, and the iris.

Choroid

The choroid is the section of the uveal tract that extends from the optic nerve to the ora serrata (where the sensory retina ends), beyond which it continues as the ciliary body [1,2]. The thickness of the choroid varies from 0.22 mm at the posterior pole to 0.10 mm near the ora serrata, at the optic nerve head, where it forms part of the optic nerve canal, and at the point of internal penetration of the vortex veins [1,2]. The uvea is supplied by the ophthalmic artery. The inner surface of the choroid is smooth and firmly attached to the retinal pigment epithelium (RPE). Its outer surface is roughened and is firmly attached to the sclera in the region of the optic nerve and where the posterior ciliary arteries and ciliary nerve enter the eye. It is also tethered to the sclera where the vortex veins leave the eyeball. This accounts for the characteristic shape of choroidal detachment (CD), which shows tethering at the site of the vortex veins and posterior ciliary arteries and ciliary nerves. Grossly, the choroid can be divided into four layers, extending from internally to externally as (1) Bruch's membrane, (2) the choriocapillaris, (3) the stroma, and (4) the suprachoroid [1]. Bruch's membrane (2–4 μm thick) is a rough, acellular, amorphous, bilamellar structure, situated between the retina and the rest of the choroid. Microscopically, Bruch's membrane consists of five layers: (1) the basement membrane of the RPE, (2) the inner collagenous zone, (3) a meshwork of elastic fibers, (4) the outer collagenous zone, and (5) the basement membrane of the choriocapillaris [4,7,8]. When a choroidal malignant melanoma penetrates through Bruch's membrane, it results in a characteristic mushroom-shaped (collar button) growth configuration.

Ciliary body

The ciliary body is continuous posteriorly with the choroid and anteriorly with the iris [see Fig. 1]. The ciliary body can be considered as a complete ring that runs around the inside of the anterior sclera. The anterior surface of the ciliary body is ridged or plicated and is called the pars plicata. The pars plicata is 2 mm in length and is composed of about 70 ciliary processes arranged radially [9]. The posterior surface of the ciliary body is smooth and flat and is called the pars plana. The pars plana is 4 mm in length and is located between pars plicata and the ora serrata. The ciliary body is made up of (1) the ciliary epithelium, (2) the ciliary stroma, and (3) the ciliary muscle. The epithelium consists of two layers of cuboidal cells that cover the inner surface of the ciliary body [1,2,4,9]. The inner layer is comprised of pigmented epithelial cells, whereas the outer layer is comprised of nonpigmented epithelial cells [9]. The ciliary stroma consists of loose connective tissue, rich in blood vessels and melanocytes, containing the embedded ciliary muscle [1]. The aqueous humor is produced in the nonpigmented epithelial layer of the ciliary body [9]. The nonpigmented epithelial cells secrete mucopolysaccharide acid, one of the main components of the vitreous [9].

Iris

The iris forms the anterior portion of the uvea. It is a thin, contractile, pigmented diaphragm with a central aperture, the pupil [see Fig. 1]. It is suspended in the aqueous humor between the cornea and the lens and divides the anterior ocular compartment (segment) into anterior and posterior chambers. The aqueous humor, formed by the ciliary processes in the posterior chamber, circulates through the pupil into the anterior chamber and exits into the sinus venous (canal of Schlemm) at the iridocorneal angle [1,2,4]. The iris consists of a stroma and two epithelial layers. The stroma consists of vascular connective tissue containing melanocytes, nerve fibers, the smooth muscle of the sphincter papillae, and the myoepithelial cells of the dilator papillae [4]. The iris pigment epithelium is continuous with the pigmented and nonpigmented layers of the ciliary body.

Retina

The retina is the sensory inner layer of the globe. The internal surface of the retina is in contact with the vitreous body and its external surface is in contact with the choroid. Grossly, the retina can be considered as having two layers: the inner layer, which is the sensory retina (ie, photoreceptors) and the first- and second-order neurons (ganglion cells) and neuroglial elements of the retina (Müller's cells, or sustentacular gliocytes); and the outer layer, which is the RPE, consisting of a single layer of cells whose nuclei are adjacent to the basal lamina

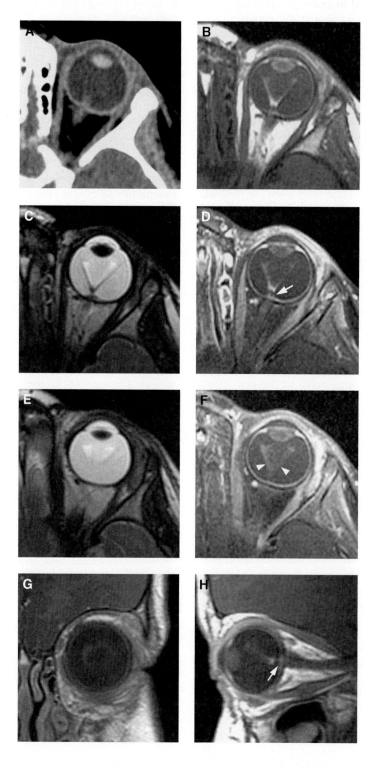

(Bruch's membrane) of the choroid [1,10,11]. The retina is very thin, measuring 0.056 mm near the disk and 0.1 mm anteriorly at the ora serrata. It is thinnest at the fovea of the macula [1]. The sensory retina extends forward from the optic disk to a point just posterior to the ciliary body. Here the nervous tissues of the retina end and its anterior edge forms a crenated wavy ring called ora serrata [1]. The RPE at the ora serrata becomes continuous with the pigmented and nonpigmented cell layers of the ciliary body and its processes [1,2]. The macula, the center of the retina, lies 3.5 mm temporal to the optic disk. The retina is attached very tightly at the margin of the optic disk and at its anterior termination at the ora serrata. It is also firmly attached to the vitreous, but loosely to the RPE and it is nourished by the choroid and the RPE [1,2]. The disk is pierced by the central retinal artery and vein. At the disk, there is complete absence of rods and cones. The disk is insensitive to light and is referred to as the "blind spot." The RPE cells are joined to each other by tight junctions. This arrangement forms a barrier, the so-called "retinal blood barrier." This limits the flow of ions and prevents diffusion of large toxic molecules from the choroid capillaries to the photoreceptors of the retina. The blood supply to the retina is from two sources: the outer lamina, including the rods and cones is supplied by the choroidal capillaries (the vessels do not enter the tissues, but tissue fluid exudes between these cells); the inner parts of the retina are supplied by the central retinal artery [1,2]. The retina depends on both of these circulations, neither of which alone is sufficient [1,2,4]. Small anastomoses occur between the branches of the posterior ciliary arteries and the central retinal artery (cilioretinal artery). The central retinal vein leaves the eyeball through the lamina cribrosa. The vein crosses the subarachnoid space and drains directly into the cavernous sinus or the superior ophthalmic vein. The retina has no lymphatic vessels.

Vitreous

The vitreous body occupies the space between the lens and retina and represents two thirds of the volume of the eye or approximately 4 mL [12]. All but 1% to 2% of the vitreous is water, bound to a fibrillar collagen meshwork of soluble proteins, some salts, and hyaluronic acid [1,2,10]. The clear, gel-like fluid that fills the vitreous chamber possesses a network of fine collagen fibrils that form scaffolding [1,2,4]. The vitreous body is the largest and simplest connective tissue present as a single structure in the human body [11]. Any insult to the vitreous body may result in a fibroproliferative reaction (eg, vitreoretinopathy of prematurity or diabetes), which can subsequently result in a tractional retinal detachment (RD) [10]. The vitreous body is bounded by the anterior and posterior hyaloid membranes. As one ages, the vitreous gel may undergo changes and start to shrink or thicken, forming strands or clumps inside the vitreous chamber, causing the so-called "floaters." Floaters are in fact tiny clumps of gel or cells inside the vitreous chamber. When the vitreous gel shrinks, it creates traction on the posterior hyaloid membrane, resulting in posterior vitreous detachment [**Figs. 2 and 3**]. The vitreous body is attached to the sensory retina, especially at the ora serrata and the margin of the optic disk [4]. It is also attached to the ciliary epithelium in the region of the pars plana [4]. The attachment of the vitreous to the lens is firm in young people and weakens with age [1,2]. During the first month of gestation, the space between the lens and the retina contains the primary vitreous. It consists of the embryonic intraocular hyaloid vascular system, embryonic connective tissue, and fibrillar meshwork. Shortly, collagen fibers and a ground substance or gel component consisting of hyaluronic acid are produced. They form the secondary vitreous and begin to replace the vascular elements of the primary vitreous [1]. By the fourteenth week of gestation, the secondary vitreous begins to fill the vitreous cavity. By the sixth month of fetal development, the cavity of the eye is filled with the secondary vitreous, which is identical to the adult vitreous. The primary vitreous is reduced to a small central space, Cloquet's canal (hyaloid canal), which runs in an S-shaped course between the optic disk and the posterior surface of the lens. During fetal life this channel contains the hyaloid artery. The artery disappears about 6 weeks before birth, and the canal

---

Fig. 2. Presumed posterior hyaloid detachment. An 18-month-old child who has leukocoria of the left eye. Retinoblastoma could not be excluded on clinical evaluation. (A) Axial CT scan shows a noncalcified lesion, presumed to be hematoma at the left optic disk. Note a faint V-shaped linear image, extending toward the optic disk. Axial unenhanced T1-weighted (B), axial T2-weighted (C), axial enhanced fat-suppressed T1-weighted (D), axial T2-weighted (E), axial enhanced fat-suppressed T1-weighted (F), coronal enhanced T1-weighted (G), and sagittal enhanced T1-weighted (H) MR images showing the detached posterior hyaloid membrane (arrowheads in F). Note that the apex of the V-shaped detachment, is connected to the optic disk by a faint ill-defined linear tissue (arrows in D and H), representing the attached part of the vitreous to the retina at the edge of the optic disk. (A–C from Mafee MF, Valvassori GE, Becker M, editors. Imaging of the head and neck. Stuttgart (Germany): Thieme; 2004; with permission.)

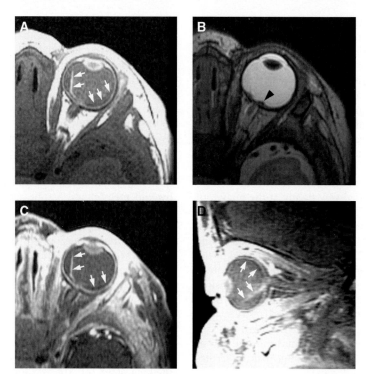

Fig. 3. Posterior hyaloid detachment. Axial unenhanced T1-weighted (*A*), axial T2-weighted (*B*), axial enhanced fat-suppressed T1-weighted (*C*), and sagittal enhanced fat-suppressed T1-weighted (*D*) MR images showing detachment of the vitreous (*arrows*). The vitreous base attachment to the retina at the optic disk is not detached. The hypointensity adjacent to the disk (*arrowhead* in *B*) is thought to be caused by hemorrhage.

becomes filled with liquid [4]. The vitreous body transmits lights, supports the posterior surface of the lens, and assists in holding the sensory retina against the RPE.

Ocular pathology

Intraocular potential spaces and ocular detachments

There are basically three potential spaces in the eye [see Fig. 1] that can accumulate fluid, causing detachment of various layers of the eyeball: (1) the posterior hyaloid space, the potential space between the base of the vitreous (posterior hyaloid membrane) and the sensory retina; (2) the subretinal space, the potential space between the sensory retina and the RPE; and (3) the suprachoroidal space, the potential space between choroid and the sclera. Another potential space is the episcleral or Tenon's space, which is between the outer surface of the sclera and inner surface of the Tenon's capsule.

Posterior hyaloid detachment

Separation of the posterior hyaloid membrane from the sensory retina is referred to as "posterior vit-

reous" or "hyaloid detachment" [1,2]. In older patients, the vitreous tends to undergo degeneration and liquefaction. Extensive vitreous liquefaction leads to posterior hyaloid detachment. Accelerated vitreous liquefaction is associated with significant myopia, surgical or nonsurgical trauma, intraocular inflammation, post laser surgery of the eye, and persistent hyperplastic primary vitreous (PHPV). On CT and MR imaging, the detached posterior hyaloid membrane can be seen as a membrane within the vitreous cavity [see Fig. 2]. The detached membrane is separated from the disk (or may be attached to the disk by a thin band) and attached at the level of ora serrata [see Figs. 2 and 3]. There may be fluid in the retrohyaloid space, which shifts its location in the lateral decubitus position.

Retinal detachment

RD occurs when the sensory retina is separated from the RPE. RD resulting from a hole or tear in the retina is referred to as "rhegmatogenous" (*rhegma* from Greek meaning to rent or rupture) RD. The sine qua non for a rhegmatogenous RD is vitreous liquefaction. Extensive vitreous liquefaction causes posterior hyaloid detachment, which in turn causes a tear at the site of vitreoretinal attachment or adhesion. The ensuing retinal break allows vitreous fluid to pass through the break into the subretinal space. Rhegmatogenous RDs are rare in pediatric patients. Most RDs in children are nonrhegmatogenous but are secondary to various ocular disease, such as retinoblastoma, PHPV, retinopathy of prematurity, Coats' disease [see Fig. 4], toxocariasis, and others. RD may be the result of retraction caused by a mass; a fibro-proliferative disease in the vitreous, such as vitreo-retinopathy of prematurity or vitreoretinopathy of diabetes mellitus; or accompanying an inflammatory process, such as *Toxocara* endophthalmitis [1,2]. Serous or exudative RD develops when the retinal-blood barrier is damaged. A breakdown of the retinal blood barrier with impairment of the RPE results in RD (nonrhegmatogenous RD). An increased fluid flow into the potential subretinal space (eg, in Coats' disease, scleritis, choroidal in-flammation, choroidal mass, other intraocular tumor, or vitreous disease entities) may result in exudative RD. Exudative fluid may be shallow or bullous. Fluid may not extend all the way to the ora serrata [Fig. 5]. In severe cases the detached retina may be so bullous as to contact the posterior lens surface [Fig. 6]. The common and uncommon causes of serous RD are summarized in Box 1. RD typically causes decreased vision. Other visual complaints, such as pain, photophobia, redness, sudden onset of tiny floating objects (floaters), and photopsia (flashes), may be present. The presence of sudden flashes of light and sudden appearance of floaters should cause serious consideration of RD. If RD is shallow, the diagnosis can be made easily with indirect ophthalmoscopy. If the retina is

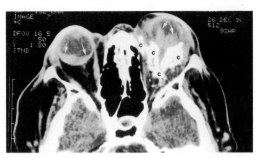

Fig. 5. Bilateral retinal detachment and orbital primary amyloidosis. Axial CT scan shows bilateral exudative retinal detachment (*arrows*). The detachment appears bullous on the left eye. The irregular calcifications (C) involving the left retrobulbar space are related to biopsy-proved amyloidosis. The cause of retinal detachment was not clear in this case.

bullously detached, however, the diagnosis may be difficult [13]. Ultrasound, CT, and MR imaging can be used to make the diagnosis. In the authors' experience, MR imaging is superior to other imaging techniques to demonstrate features that could

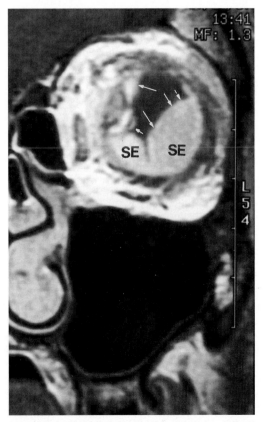

Fig. 6. Retinal detachment. Coronal enhanced T1-weighted MR image shows the characteristic corrugated retinal folds (*arrows*) on coronal view. The subretinal exudate (SE) signal was the same on unenhanced T1-weighted MR images.

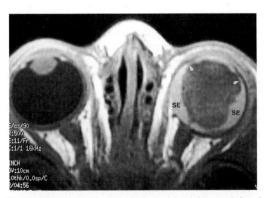

Fig. 4. Retinal detachment. Enhanced axial T1-weighted MR image in a child who has Coats' disease shows an exudative retinal detachment of the left eye. Note subretinal exudates (SE), which had the same signal intensity on unenhanced axial MR image. The detached sensory retina is limited at the ora serrata (*arrows*) and at the optic disk. The increased intensity of the left vitreous is related to protein leaking into the vitreous from abnormal retinal vessels.

differentiate different causes of RD. Exudative RD is characterized by shifting subretinal fluid, which assumes a dependent position beneath the retina. On CT and MR imaging, the appearance of RD varies with the amount of exudate, presence of hemorrhage, and organization of the subretinal materials. In a section taken at the level of the optic nerve disk, RD is seen with a characteristic V-shaped configuration with the apex at the optic disk and its extremities toward the ora serrata [see Fig. 4]. When total RD is present and the entire vitreous cavity is ablated, the leaves of the detached retina may touch at the center of the eye and appear as a folding membrane extending from the optic disk to the posterior surface of the lens, simulating

Cloquet's canal. The MR imaging signal intensity of subretinal fluid depends on the protein content and presence or absence of hemorrhage. The subretinal fluid of an exudative RD is rich in protein, giving higher CT attenuation values and stronger MR imaging signal intensities (on T1-weighted MR images) [see Fig. 4] than those seen in the subretinal fluid (transudate) of a rhegmatogenous detachment. In rhegmatogenous RD, produced by a retinal tear and subsequent ingress of vitreous fluid into the subretinal space, the signal of subretinal transudate is almost isointense to vitreous, making visualization of detached retina more difficult. RD is seen on coronal CT and MR images as a characteristic folding membrane, representing corrugated retinal folds [Fig. 6].

Choroidal detachment and choroidal effusion

CD is caused by the accumulation of fluid (serous CD) or blood (hemorrhagic CD) in the potential suprachoroidal space [1,2,10,14–16]. Serous CD frequently occurs after intraocular surgery, penetrating ocular trauma, or inflammatory choroidal disorders [14]. Ocular hypotony is the essential underlying cause of serous CD. Ocular hypotony may be the result of ocular inflammatory diseases (uveitis, scleritis); accidental perforation of the eye; ocular surgery; or intensive glaucoma therapy. The pressure within the suprachoroidal space is determined by the intraocular pressure, the intracapillary blood pressure, and the oncotic pressure exerted by the plasma protein colloids [17]. The capillaries of the choroid are fenestrated and these openings are covered by diaphragms, which permit the relatively free exchange of material between the choriocapillaris and the surrounding tissues [18]. Ocular hypotony results in increased permeability of the choriocapillaris, and this in turn leads to the transudation of fluid from the choroidal vasculature into the uveal tissue causing diffuse swelling of the entire choroid (choroidal effusion). As the edema of the choroid increases, fluid may accumulate in the potential suprachoroidal space, resulting in serous or exudative CD [14–16]. Other causes of choroidal effusion include inflammatory disorders of the eye, myxedema, photocoagulation, retinal cryopexy, Vogt-Koyanagi-Harada syndrome, nanophthalmos, and idiopathic uveal effusion syndrome. Nanophthalmos is an autosomal-recessive disorder in which there is bilateral short axial length globes, normal-sized lenses, and thick sclerae. As a result of scleral thickening, the scleral outflow channels and transscleral passage of vortex veins become impaired. This can lead to choroidal congestion, choroidal thickening, and eventually choroidal effusion [see Fig. 7]. The management of choroidal effusion in nanophthalmos and idiopathic choroidal effu-

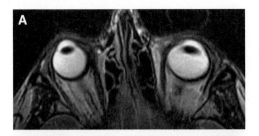

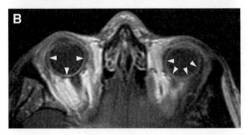

Fig. 7. Nanophthalmos and associated choroidal effusion. Axial T2-weighted (*A*) and enhanced axial T1-weighted (*B*) MR images. Note bilateral short axial length globes and marked thickened sclerae (*A*), and increased uveal enhancement (*arrowheads*), the left being greater than the right.

sion is surgical and consists of sclerotomy (scleral window operation) to decompress the vortex veins [13]. Hemorrhagic CD is a serious condition that may be associated with permanent loss of vision [19]. Both localized and massive choroidal hemorrhage may occur as a complication of most forms of ocular surgery and ocular trauma. Choroidal hemorrhage may occur in association with hemoglobinopathies in patients receiving anticoagulant therapy, or spontaneously [19]. Intraoperative choroidal hemorrhage may progress to expulsion of intraocular tissues (expulsive choroidal hemorrhage) [19]. Clinically, the CD appears as a smooth gray–brown elevation of the choroid, extending from the ciliary body to the posterior segment [14,15]. Ophthalmoscopic visualization of the fundus may be precluded by hyphema (blood in the anterior chamber) or vitreous hemorrhage. Even when the other ocular media are clear, in pigmented eyes it is difficult to differentiate between serous and hemorrhagic CD with ophthalmoscopy [14,15]. Localized choroidal hemorrhage may be mistaken for a choroidal melanoma, particularly when it presents as a discrete, dark posterior ocular mass [19]. Ultrasonography can be very useful for the diagnosis of CD, however, ultrasonography has certain limitations in examin-

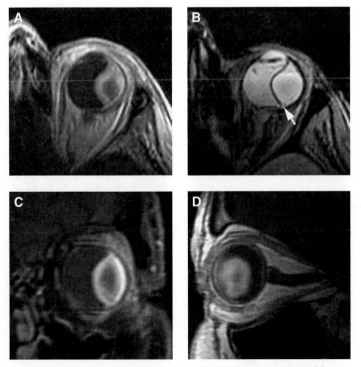

Fig. 8. Hemorrhagic choroidal detachment. Axial T1-weighted (*A*), axial T2-weighted (*B*), coronal T1-weighted (*C*), and sagittal T1-weighted (*D*) MR images showing a chronic hemorrhagic choroidal detachment. Note that the detached choroid is restricted at the expected level of the vortex vein or posterior ciliary artery (*arrow*). Note that the detached choroid extends to the ciliary body.

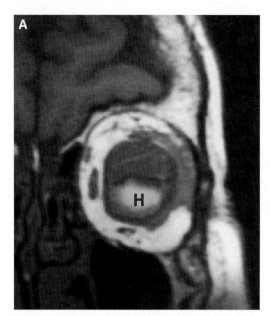
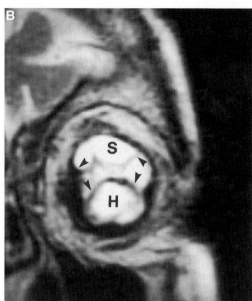

Fig. 9. Serous and hemorrhagic choroidal detachment. Coronal T1-weighted (*A*) and T2-weighted (*B*) MR images showing an inferior hemorrhagic (H) and superior serous (S) choroidal detachment. Note detached choroid (*arrows*), which is restricted at the expected level of vortex veins.

ing traumatized eyes. The appearance of serous CD and limited or diffuse hemorrhagic CD on CT has been described [14]. It appears as a smooth, dome-shaped, semilunar area of variable attenuation values. The degree of CT attenuation depends on the cause but is generally greater with inflammatory disorders of the eyeball. Hemorrhagic CD appears as either a low or high mound-like area of high density on CT. In a fresh hemorrhagic CD, the choroid and hematoma are isodense. In chronic hematoma, however, it may be possible to differentiate detached choroid and suprachoroidal fluid accumulation [see Figs. 8 and 9]. Serial CT, MR imaging, and ultrasonography reveal diminishing size over a period of several weeks or months. MR imaging is an excellent method to evaluate the eye in patients who have CD, particularly if ultrasonography or CT in conjunction with the clinical examination has not provided sufficient information [1]. On MR imaging, a limited choroidal hematoma appears as a focal, well-demarcated, smooth dome-shaped or lenticular mass [Fig. 8]. It is important to realize that this characteristic configuration usually does not change as the hematoma ages [16]. A decrease in the size of the choroidal hematoma, however, may be observed. Multiple lesions may be present [see Fig. 9]. The signal intensity of choroidal hematoma depends on its age. Within the first 48 hours, the hematoma is isointense to slightly hypointense relative to the normal vitreous on T1-weighted MR images but is markedly hypointense on T2-weighted MR images. After few days, its signal intensity changes,

being relatively hyperintense on T1-weighted and hypointense on T2-weighted MR images. Chronic choroidal hematoma (3 weeks or older) become hyperintense on T1-weighted and T2-weighted MR images [see **Figs. 8 and 9**]. Serous CD and choroidal effusion have a different MR appearance compared with choroidal hematoma. The fluid in the suprachoroidal space in serous CD is often hypodense on CT, and its MR appearance is that of an exudate

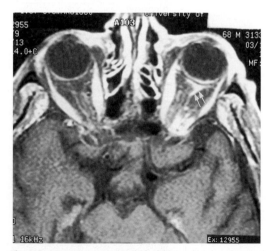

Fig. 10. Herpes zoster ophthalmitis. Axial enhanced fat-suppressed T1-weighted MR image shows abnormal enhancement along the left optic nerve sheath (*arrows*). Note also increased enhancement of left posterior globe.

[Fig. 9]. At times, the appearance of CD and RD may be confused. Scleral attachments of the vortex veins restrict further detachment of the choroid beyond the anchoring point of the vortex veins, however, and similarly beyond the short posterior ciliary arteries and nerves. This restriction usually results in a characteristic appearance of the leaves of the detached choroid, which unlike the detached retinal leaves do not extend to the region of the optic nerve [see **Figs. 8 and 9**]. In addition, unlike the detached leaves of the retina, which end at the ora serrata, the detached choroid can extend to the ciliary body and also result in ciliary detachment [see **Fig. 10**].

Ocular inflammatory disorders

The eye may be affected by known or idiopathic inflammatory processes. A host of infectious diseases may affect the globe. Viral infections include herpes simplex, herpes zoster [**Fig. 10**], cytomegalovirus [**Fig. 11**], rubella, rubeola, mumps, variola, varicella, and infectious mononucleosis [1]. Bacterial diseases include tuberculosis, syphilis, Lyme disease, brucellosis, leprosy, cat-scratch disease, *Escherichia coli* infection, and other agents.

Fungal infections, particularly candidiasis, may involve the globes in diabetic and immunocompromised patients [1]. Parasitic infections, particularly *Toxocara canis*, cause granulomatous chorioretinitis with an eosinophilic abscess.

Scleritis

The sclera may be the site of a number of inflammatory or noninflammatory processes. Episcleritis is a relatively common idiopathic inflammation of a thin layer of loose connective tissue between the sclera and the conjunctiva. Episcleritis is usually self-limited and resolves within 1 or 2 weeks [20].

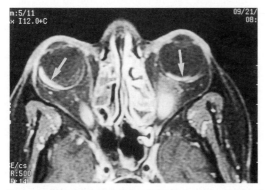

Fig. 11. Cytomegalovirus retinitis. Axial enhanced fat-suppressed T1-weighted MR image shows marked enhancement of posterior globes (*arrows*) in this immunocompromised patient who has bilateral cytomegalovirus retinitis.

Imaging is not indicated in episcleritis. In contrast to episcleritis, scleritis is a rare condition, and a more serious disorder. Scleritis can occur as an idiopathic condition (50%) or in association with rheumatoid arthritis, other connective tissue diseases, or with a group of other disorders, such as Wegener's granulomatosis, relapsing polychondritis, inflammatory bowel disease, Crohn's disease, Cogan's syndrome, and sarcoidosis [1]. In scleritis, histopathology may demonstrate granulomatous or nongranulomatous inflammation, vasculitis, and scleral necrosis [20]. Histopathologically, posterior scleritis is classified into two forms: nodular and diffuse. The term "posterior scleritis" refers to scleral inflammation behind the equator. Patients who have posterior scleritis may develop exudative RD, disk swelling, and CD [20,21]. Scleritis may be associated with uveitis (iritis, choroiditis) and increased intraocular pressure. Inflammatory debris may block scleral emissary veins, resulting in elevated episcleral venous pressure and hence elevated intraocular pressure. Ciliary body detachment adjacent to active anterior scleritis may cause angle closure glaucoma. If scleritis is associated with uveitis, the trabecular meshwork may be clogged with inflammatory debris and cells, causing glaucoma. On CT scans and MR images, posterior scleritis results in thickening of the sclera [**Fig. 12**]. There may be associated thickening of Tenon's capsule (sclerotenonitis) and secondary serous RD or serous CD. In general, it is easier to see these changes related to posterior scleritis on CT scans rather than MR images. Posterior nodular scleritis is a focal or zonal necrotizing granulomatous inflammation of the sclera. On imaging this entity may mimic choroidal malignant melanoma or ocular lymphoma.

Uveitis

Inflammation of the uvea (uveitis) may be limited to the anterior uvea (iritis), ciliary body (cyclitis), the posterior uvea, or the choroid (choroiditis, posterior uveitis). Posterior cyclitis (pars planitis) is referred to as "intermediate uveitis." Inflammatory diseases of the uvea are seldom limited to this vascularized layer of the eye. The sclera and retina are usually involved [1]. Posterior uveitis may be focal, multifocal, diffuse choroiditis, chorioretinitis, or neurouveitis [22]. The etiology of uveitis is often unknown. Traumatic iridocyclitis is the most common cause of anterior uveitis. Most intermediate uveitis is idiopathic [22]. The most common causes of panuveitis are idiopathic and sarcoidosis. Uveitis may be seen in patients who have juvenile rheumatoid arthritis, seronegative spondyloarthropathies, and herpetic keratouveitis. Uveitis may be caused by a specific organism, such as *Toxoplasma*. Other causes include bacterial posterior uveitis including Whipple's disease; viral uveitis

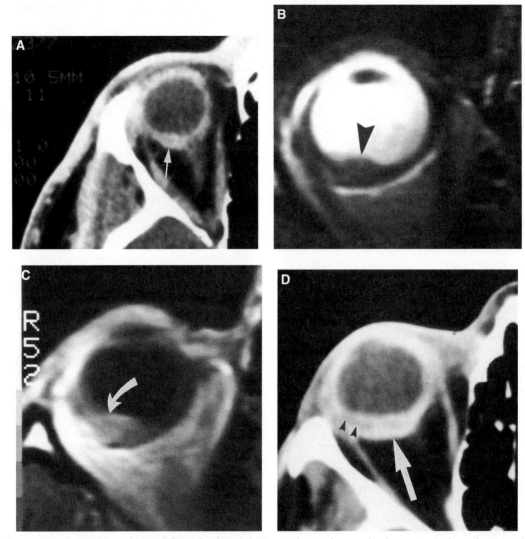

Fig. 12. Posterior nodular scleritis. (*A*) Axial enhanced CT scan shows abnormal enhancement along the posterior aspect of the right globe (*arrow*). Axial T2-weighted (*B*) and axial enhanced T1-weighted (*C*) MR images showing a mass-like lesion (*arrowhead* in *B* and *arrow* in *C*) compatible with posterior nodular scleritis. This CT and MR imaging appearance may not be differentiated from a choroidal mass. Patient responded well to a course of steroid therapy. (*D*) Enhanced axial CT scan in another patient who has necrotizing keratitis and scleritis showing thickening of the Tenon's capsule (*arrow*), fluid in the episcleral space (*arrowheads*), and marked thickening and increased enhancement of the sclera.

(cytomegalovirus, herpes simplex, Coxsackie virus); fungal uveitis; and parasitic uveitis. Some forms of uveitis, such as sarcoidosis, Vogt-Koyanagi-Harada syndrome, and Behçet's syndrome, have strong ethnic association. Vogt-Koyanagi-Harada syndrome is an idiopathic bilateral chronic granulomatous uveitis, with exudative choroidal effusion and nonrheg-matogenous RD associated with alopecia, vitiligo, hearing problems, meningeal signs, pleocytosis in the cerebrospinal fluid, and poliosis. Behçet's syndrome is a multisystem vasculitis of unknown cause. Patients usually present with a history of oral and genital ulcerations. Vogt-Koyanagi-Harada

is a cell-mediated autoimmune disease. It is often a self-limiting disease. Sympathetic uveitis is a rare bilateral autoimmune-related uveitis that develops after penetrating injury to the eye. Larval uveitis results from ingestion of the eggs of the nematode *T canis* or *Toxocara cati*. Imaging is not indicated in classic nontraumatic anterior uveitis. Patients who have granulomatous uveitis or posterior uveitis of unclear cause may benefit from ultrasound, CT, or MR imaging to assess the degree of choroidal or scleral thickening, masses (eg, abscess), and to evaluate for the presence of RD, choroidal effusion, or intraocular foreign bodies, particularly in patients

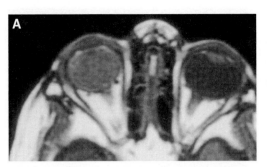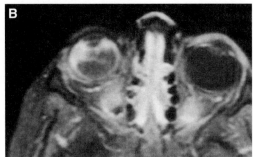

Fig. 13. Granulomatous uveitis. Axial T1-weighted (*A*) and enhanced fat-suppressed axial T1-weighted (*B*) MR images in a 3-year-old child showing marked enhancement of the right globe, predominantly adjacent to the ciliary body. Note increased intensity of the vitreous in precontrast T1-weighted image (*A*), representing leakage of protein into the vitreous or associated vitreous inflammation.

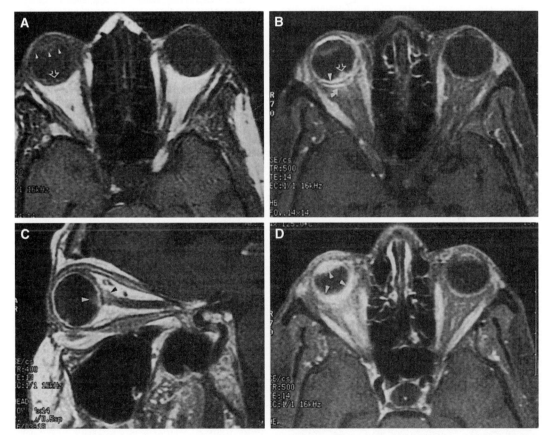

Fig. 14. Ocular sarcoidosis panuveitis. (*A*) Unenhanced axial T1-weighted (500/13 TR/TE) MR image shows nodular thickening of the posterior aspect of the right globe (*arrow*) and thickening of the anterior segment (*arrowheads*) of the right globe. (*B*) Enhanced axial fat-suppressed T1-weighted (500/13 TR/TE) MR image shows nodular enhancement of the posterior aspect of the right globe (*arrowhead* and *open arrow*) related to granulomatous involvement of the choroid. Note enhancement of the anterior segment of the right globe. Notice abnormal enhancement of Tenon's capsule (*curved arrow*). (*C*) Enhanced sagittal T1-weighted (400/13 TR/TE) MR image shows granuloma at the optic disk (*white arrowhead*) and involvement of the optic nerve (*black arrowhead*). (*D*) Enhanced axial fat-suppressed T1-weighted (500/14 TR/TE) MR image shows enhancement of markedly thickened uveal tract (*arrowheads*). (*From* Mafee MF, Dorodi S, Pai E. Saroidosis of the eye, orbit, and central nervous system. Role of MR imaging. Radiol Clin North Am 1999;37:74.)

who have media opacities [Figs. 13 and 14]. Optic disk enhancement on MR imaging and CT scans may be seen in patients who have pseudotumor cerebri [Fig. 15], simulating posterior uveitis, uveoneurol retinitis of cat-scratch disease, and retinal and choroidal tumors.

Endophthalmitis

Endophthalmitis refers to an intraocular infectious or noninfectious inflammatory process predominantly involving the vitreous cavity or anterior chamber. It is a serious complication following intraocular surgery, nonsurgical trauma, or systemic infection [23]. The visual outcome despite aggressive treatment in many cases remains poor. In exogenous endophthalmitis, the organisms gain access to eye by surgical or nonsurgical trauma (mostly from patient's lid and conjunctival flora), or may gain access to the eye hematogenously (endogenous endophthalmitis) from an infectious focus, such as endocarditis, urinary tract or bowel infections, or an infected intravenous line or shunt. A predisposing factor may be present, such as prematurity, leukemia, lymphoma, disseminated carcinoma, drug abuse, immunocompromise, and long-term use of corticosteroids [23]. Phacoanaphylactic endophthalmitis is a granulomatous infection that results from autoimmunity to exposed lens protein. In endogenous bacterial and fungal endophthalmitis, septic emboli are lodged in the choriocapillaris and retinal arterioles. Bruch's membrane is disrupted and organisms gain access into the retina and vitreous. The organisms most frequently isolated in endophthalmitis are *Staphylococcus epidermidis*, *Staphylococcus aureus*, streptococcal species, and *Candida*. Parasitic granulomatosis refers to ocular inflammation as a result of infec-

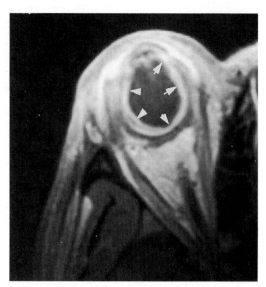

Fig. 16. Endophthalmitis. Axial enhanced T1-weighted MR image shows marked thickening and enhancement of the entire uveal tract (*arrows*).

tion with helminthic parasite. The most common of these are *T canis* or *T cati*, *Cysticercus cellulosae*, and microfilariae of *Onchocerca volvulus*. Toxocariasis result in granuloma formation in the posterior pole or periphery, and endophthalmitis. Cysticercosis may occur anywhere in the eye or around the eye. The CT and MR imaging findings in endophthalmitis include increased density of the vitreous on CT and increased signal intensity of the vitreous on T1-weighted and flair MR images because of increased protein from leaking retinal or choroidal vessels. The uvea may be thickened and demonstrates increased enhancement or focal enhancement (abscess) [Fig. 16]. Associated CD, RD, and posterior vitreous detachment may be delineated on CT and MR imaging.

Ocular calcifications

Calcification is commonly found in normal and abnormal ocular tissues. The presence of calcifications on CT scans can be used to correctly diagnose the type of pathology [Figs. 17–19] [24–26]. Idiopathic scleral calcification is seen in many patients older than 70 years of age. CT scan shows these calcified plaques near the insertions of lateral and medial rectus muscles. The calcified plaques may be in the posterior aspect of the sclera. Calcification may occur at the level of the ciliary body or in the choroid. Ciliary body calcification may be seen after trauma; after inflammation [see Fig. 17]; or in teratoid medulloepithelioma of the ciliary body. Choroidal calcification often follows severe intraocular inflammation or trauma. Choroidal osteoma

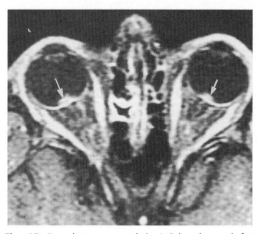

Fig. 15. Pseudotumor cerebri. Axial enhanced fat-suppressed T1-weighted MR image in a patient who has pseudotumor cerebri showing abnormal enhancement at the level of both optic discs (*arrows*).

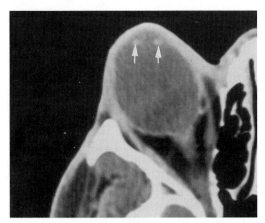

Fig. 17. Axial CT scan shows enlarged right globe caused by axial myopia. Note calcification of ciliary body (*arrows*). Lens has been removed.

is an unusual but distinct cause of choroidal calcification. The osteoma is a rare, well-defined, benign tumor (choristoma) that is found mainly in otherwise healthy young women [24]. It typically arises in the choroid adjacent to the optic nerve head of one or both eyes [Fig. 18]. Detection of calcification plays an important role in the diagnosis of malignant intraocular tumors, such as retinoblastoma and medulloepithelioma (see articles on retinoblastoma and medulloepithelioma elsewhere in this issue).

In published histopathologic series, calcium depositions have been seen to occur in necrotic areas of 87% to 95% of retinoblastoma. CT scan demonstrates calcification in more than 90% of retinoblastoma [1,2]. CT demonstration of calcification may be helpful for differentiating retinoblastoma from PHPV, retinopathy of prematurity, Coats' disease, and a variety of other nonspecific causes of leukocoria [1,2]. In children younger than 3 years of age, CT detection of appropriate intraocular calcification suggests that retinoblastoma is the most

likely diagnosis. In children older than 3 years of age, however, detection of calcification has less differential value, because some other entities including PHPV, retinopathy of prematurity, and Coats' disease can also produce calcification in older children [24]. Calcification is often absent in PHPV. In older patients, however, calcification may be found in the crystalline lens or focally in a totally detached retina. Retinopathy of prematurity is a bilateral ocular disorder resulting in abnormal proliferation of fibrovascular tissue in the retina of premature infants who previously received oxygen therapy. The abnormal tissue extends into the vitreous cavity where it causes tractional RD. Calcification in the lens, choroid, and retrolental tissue has been reported in children who have late stage of this disease [24]. Coats' disease is a unilateral exudative RD that mainly affects boys between 18 months and 18 years of age. The disease is an idiopathic congenital disorder of the retinal vessels (telangiectases). Abnormal retinal vessels can occur either in the periphery or the central retina; leakage of lipid-rich serum from telangiectatic vessels into the subretinal space results in RD [see Fig. 4]. The

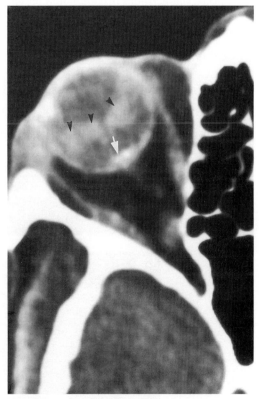

Fig. 19. Chronic retinal detachment. Axial CT scan shows retinal detachment. Note calcification at the optic disk (*arrow*). The increased thickening of the detached retina (*arrowheads*) is related to reactive retinal gliosis.

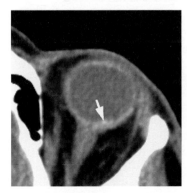

Fig. 18. Choroidal osteoma. Axial CT scan shows a calcified mass, compatible with presumed choroidal osteoma (*arrow*).

retina may be shallowly detached or become bulously detached. Patients who have Coats' disease occasionally may have calcification in the retina. This calcification may be submacular and result from metaplasia of the RPE [2,24]. RPE is capable of metaplastic calcification or bone formation [Fig. 19]. Calcification may also be detected on CT in patients who have microphthamos with or without colobomatous cyst. The calcification in these eyes most likely occurs in the choristomatous glial tissue [24]. Retinal astrocytic hamartoma is another lesion that may cause retinal calcification [2]. These hamartomas most frequently occur in tuberous sclerosis, but also may be noted in neurofibromatosis. Cytomegalovirus retinitis is a common infection in patients who have AIDS [see Fig. 11]. In cytomegalovirus retinitis, calcification may be seen in the necrotic portion of the retina, or in areas of healed retina [24]. Retinal drusen is a common cause of calcification of the RPE. Drusen are well-defined excrescences that form under the RPE in aging eyes, and are often associated with age-related macular degeneration. Retinal drusen are very small and cannot be visualized by CT scanning. Subretinal neovascular membranes are fibrovascular proliferations that arise from the choroid and extend into the subretinal space, causing serous and hemorrhagic RDs. Numerous condi-

tions may result in subretinal neovascular membranes, but age-related macular degeneration is the most common cause of subretinal neovascular membranes. Long-standing neovascular membranes may become calcified.

Drusen of the optic nerve are acellular accretions of hyaline-like material that occur on or near the surface of the optic disk. They are often seen in the prelaminar optic nerve. When drusen affect the papilla, the optic nerve head is elevated and shows blurred disk margins. Unlike retinal drusen, CT scans can readily detect optic disk drusen. Trauma in one series [24] was the single most common cause of ocular calcification. The calcification typically occurs many years after the initial trauma, when the damaged globes are in varying stages of atrophy or phthisis.

Ocular tumors

Most primary and metastatic ocular neoplasms in adults involve the uveal tract and in particular the choroid. Malignant melanoma is the most common tumor to involve the uvea [25–30]. Most primary ocular neoplasms in children, however, involve the retina. Retinoblastoma is the most common tumor to involve the retina (see the article on retinoblastoma and simulating lesions elsewhere

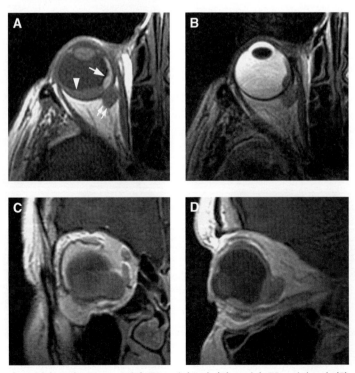

Fig. 20. Malignant choroidal melanoma. Axial T1-weighted (*A*), axial T2-weighted (*B*), coronal enhanced T1-weighted (*C*), and sagittal enhanced T1-weighted (*D*) MR images showing a plaquoid choroidal melanoma (*large arrow*), subretinal exudate (*arrowhead*), and extraocular extension of tumor (*small arrows*).

in this issue) [31–33]. Retinal astrocytic hamartoma is another rare lesion involving the retina. These hamartomas most frequently occur in tuberous sclerosis, but also may be found in neurofibromatosis. On pathologic examination, these hamartomas show focal benign astrocytic proliferation that usually contains calcium [24].

Medulloepithelioma is an embryonic neoplasm derived from primitive neuroepithelium, presenting as a mass behind the pupil and iris [33]. It typically arises from the ciliary body epithelium, but may also occur as a posterior mass in the retina or optic nerve (see the article on medulloepithelioma of the ciliary body and optic nerve elsewhere in this issue) [33,34].

Malignant uveal melanoma

Malignant uveal melanomas are the most common primary intraocular tumor in adults. Some of these tumors may originate from pre-existing nevi [30]. Choroidal hemangioma, choroidal nevi, CD, choroidal cysts, neurofibroma and schwannoma of the uvea, uveal leiomyoma, ciliary body adenoma and adenocarcinoma, medulloepithelioma, juvenile xanthogranuloma, RD, disciform degeneration of the macula, and metastatic tumors are some of the benign and malignant lesions that

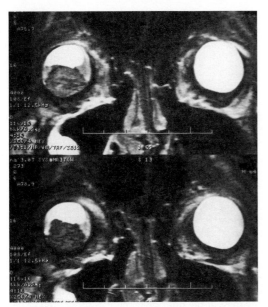

Fig. 21. Malignant choroidal melanoma. Coronal T2-weighted MR images showing a large mound-shaped choroidal melanoma (*arrows*). The MR images were obtained on a 3-T MR imaging unit using quadrature head coil.

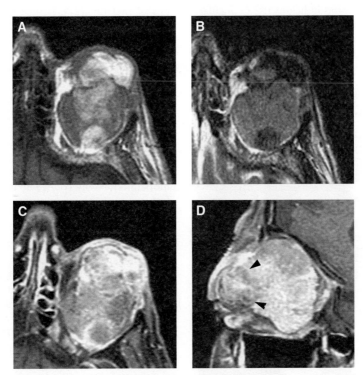

Fig. 22. Presumed ocular melanoma. Unenhanced axial T1-weighted (*A*), axial T2-weighted (*B*), enhanced axial (*C*), and sagittal T1-weighted (*D*) MR images showing an enhancing mass within the left globe (*arrowheads*) and a large retrobulbar mass. Eye examination showed a large intraocular mass. The patient was found to have multiple liver masses.

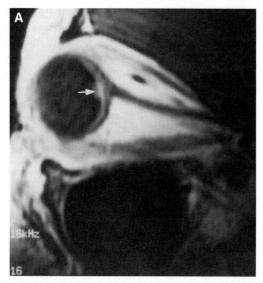

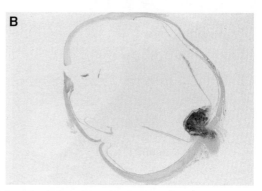

Fig. 23. Melanocytoma and melanoma of the optic disk. (*A*) Sagittal T1-weighted MR image shows a mass (*arrow*) at the optic disk. (*B*) photomicrograph of the eye showing the mass at the optic disk. This was considered to be a melanoma arising from a melanocytoma.

may be confused with malignant uveal melanoma [27–30,34]. Because of their anatomic location, tumors of the uveal tract are not accessible to biopsy without intraocular surgery. Consequently, the diagnosis must often be made on the basis of clinical examination and judicious use of ancillary diagnostic procedures, such as fluorescein angiography, ultrasonography, CT, and MR imaging. This article only considers the role of MR imaging in

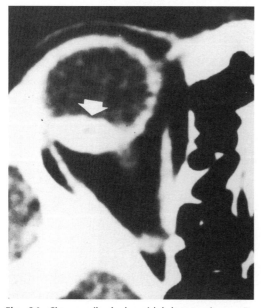

Fig. 24. Circumscribed choroidal hemangioma. Enhanced CT scan shows an intensely enhancing choroidal hemangioma (*arrows*).

the diagnosis of uveal melanoma. The MR imaging techniques for ocular lesions have been described in several prior publications [1,2,30]. The MR imaging characteristics of melanotic lesions are thought to be related to the paramagnetic properties of melanin [27]. Unlike most tumors, melanomas have short T1 and T2 relaxation time values. Most uveal melanomas appear as areas of high signal intensity on T1- and proton-weighted MR images [Fig. 20]. On T2-weighted MR images, melanomas appear as areas of moderately low signal intensity [Figs. 20 and 21]. The tumor may be dome-shaped [Fig. 21], mushroom-shaped, plaquoid [see Fig. 20], ring-shaped, or diffuse. Although in general the paramagnetic property of melanin plays an important role in MR imaging signal characteristics of melanomas, the histologic features of tumors undoubtedly contribute to their MR imaging features [30]. Melanomas are often arranged in tightly cohesive bundles and are highly cellular (short T2 relaxation time). Necrosis and hemorrhage are not uncommon [1,2,27,30]. At times, uveal melanomas may appear partially or completely hyperintense on T2-weighted MR images. Exudative or hemorrhagic RD may be present [see Fig. 20]. Extensive extraocular extension may be present even in the presence of a small intraocular malignant melanoma [Fig. 22]. Gadolinium diethylenetriamine pentaacetic acid contrast material is very useful in the diagnosis of uveal melanomas, certain ocular pathology, and, in particular, for evaluation of optic nerve and retrobulbar extension of ocular tumors [see Fig. 20]. Uveal melanomas demonstrate moderate enhance-

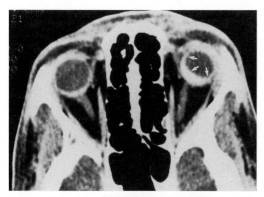

Fig. 25. Diffuse choroidal hemangioma. Enhanced CT scan shows a diffuse choroidal hemangioma (*arrows*).

ment on postgadolinium T1-weighted MR images [see **Fig. 20**].

Melanocytoma is a deeply pigmented benign tumor that may occur in the uvea and in the substance of the optic nerve. Approximately 50% of melanocytomas develop in blacks, whereas the incidence of malignant uveal melanoma in blacks is less than 1%. The MR imaging appearance of melanocytoma is similar to uveal melanoma [**Fig. 23**].

Choroidal hemangioma

Choroidal hemangiomas are congenital vascular hamartomas typically seen in middle-aged to elderly individuals [35,36]. Two different forms have been reported: a circumscribed or solitary type not associated with other abnormalities; and a diffuse angiomatosis often associated with facial nevus flammeus or variations of the Sturge-Weber syndrome [1–3,6,37]. The solitary choroidal hemangioma is confined to choroid, shows distinct margins, and characteristically lies posterior to the equator of the globe [36]. It is typically seen as a tumor located in the juxtapapillary or macular region of the fundus [36]. In contrast, the hemangioma associated with Sturge-Weber syndrome is a diffuse process that may involve the choroid, ciliary body, iris, and, occasionally, nonuveal tissues, such as the episclera, conjunctiva, and limbus [37]. CT, including dynamic CT, has been shown to be useful for the diagnosis of choroidal hemangioma [**Figs. 24 and 25**] [36,38]. MR imaging has been shown to be superior to CT for evaluation of uveal melanomas, choroidal hemangioma, and simulating lesions [1,2,27,37,38]. On T1-weighted MR images, the choroidal hemangiomas appear as isointense to slightly hypertense lesions with respect to the vitreous. They appear hyperintense on T2-weighted MR images [**Fig. 26**], so they become isointense to vitreous on these pulse sequences. They demonstrate intense contrast enhancement on enhanced T1-weighted MR images [**Figs. 26 and 27**].

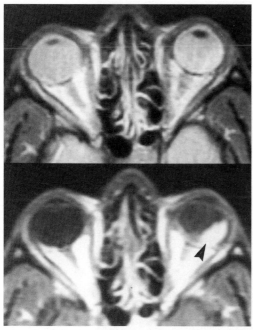

Fig. 26. Choroidal hemangioma. Proton-weighted (*top*) and enhanced T1-weighted (*bottom*) MR images showing an intensely enhancing choroidal hemangioma (*arrowhead*).

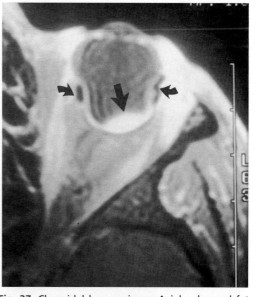

Fig. 27. Choroidal hemangioma. Axial enhanced fat-suppressed T1-weighted MR image shows an intensely enhancing choroidal hemangioma (*straight arrow*). Note scleral buckling (*curved arrows*) for the repair of retinal detachment. The cause of retinal detachment was not clear until MR imaging was performed.

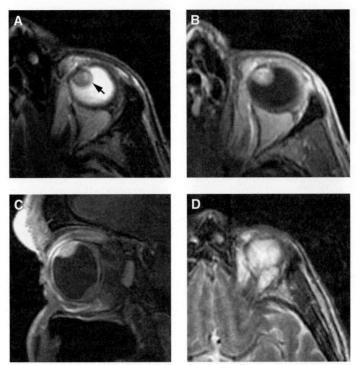

Fig. 28. Ocular metastasis. Axial T2-weighted (*A*), axial enhanced fat-suppressed T1-weighted (*B*), sagittal enhanced fat-suppressed T1-weighted (*C*), and post–proton beam treatment axial T2-weighted (*D*) MR images showing a mass (*arrow*) compatible with biopsy-proven metastatic hypernephroma. Note satisfactory response following proton beam treatment (*D*).

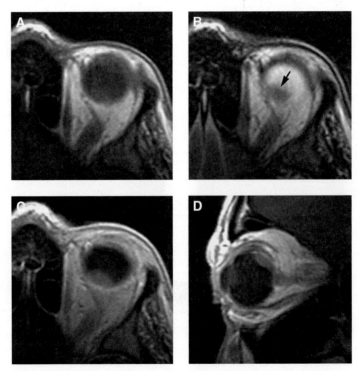

Fig. 29. Ocular metastasis. Axial T1-weighted (*A*), axial T2-weighted (*B*), enhanced axial (*C*), and sagittal T1-weighted (*D*) MR imaging showing a metastatic mass (*arrow*) from primary malignant thymoma.

Uveal metastases

Uveal metastasis can be confused clinically and radiologically with uveal melanoma. Embolic malignant cells reach the globe by means of the short posterior ciliary arteries. The route of spread may be the reason why most of the metastases involve the posterior half of the globe [27]. The most common sources of secondary tumor within the eye are the breast and lung. Both eyes may be affected in about one third of the cases. Signal intensity of uveal melanomas and uveal metastases may be similar [Figs. 28 and 29].

Other uveal tumors

Choroidal lymphoma and leukemic infiltration of the uveal tract can be mistaken for choroidal tumor. The process often is bilateral. On MR imaging its signal characteristics are similar to uveal melanoma

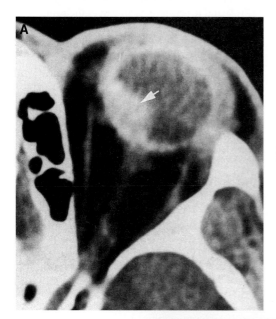
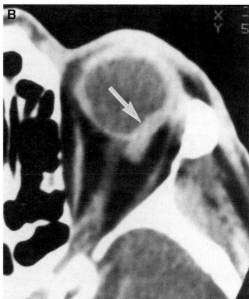
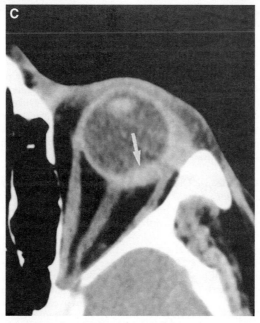

Fig. 30. Choroidal hematoma, simulating choroidal melanoma. (*A*) Axial CT scan shows a hyperdense mass (*arrow*) compatible with choroidal hematoma. (*B*) Axial CT scan shows a hyperdense mass (*arrow*) compatible with choroidal melanoma. Note extraocular extension of this melanoma. (*C*) Enhanced axial CT scan shows focal thickening of the eyeball caused by a choroidal melanoma.

[27]. Neurofibroma and schwannoma of the choroid and ciliary body, adenoma and adenocarcinoma of the ciliary body, leiomyoma of the ciliary body, and other rare lesions can also be confused with uveal melanoma on MR imaging [1,2,27].

Choroidal hematoma

Choroidal hematoma, CD (serous and hemorrhagic), and posterior scleritis may simulate choroidal melanoma, particularly on CT scans [Fig. 30].

Summary

Since the development of CT and MR imaging, significant progress has been made in ophthalmic imaging. As the technology advanced and MR imaging units improved their ability in term of spatial resolution, the role of MR imaging in ophthalmic imaging has increased accordingly. This article considers the role of MR and CT imaging in the diagnosis of selected pathologies of the eye.

Acknowledgments

The authors are grateful to Dr. Kiarash Mohajer for helpful literature research, Aura Smith for secretarial assistance, and Yasir Aich for technical support.

References

[1] Mafee MF. The eye. In: Som PM, Curtin HD, editors. Head and neck imaging. 4th edition. St. Louis (MO): Mosby; 2003. p. 441–527.

[2] Mafee MF. The eye and orbit. In: Mafee MF, Valvassori GE, Becker M, editors. Imaging of the head and neck. 2nd edition. Stuttgart (Germany): Thieme; 2005. p. 137–294.

[3] Warwich R, Williams PL. Gray's anatomy. 35th British edition. Philadelphia: WB Saunders; 1973.

[4] Snell RS, Lemp MA, editors. Clinical anatomy of the eye. Boston: Blackwell Scientific; 1989.

[5] Reech MF, Wobij JL, Wirtschapter JD. Ophthalmic anatomy: a manual with some clinical applications. San Francisco: American Academy of Ophthalmology; 1981.

[6] Mafee MF, Putterman A, Valvassori GE, et al. Orbital space occupying lesions: role of computed tomography an magnetic resonance imaging. An analysis of 145 cases. Radiol Clin North Am 1987;25:529–59.

[7] Rtumin U. Fundus appearance in normal eye. I. The choroid. Am J Ophthalmol 1967;64:821–57.

[8] Nakaizumi Y. The ultrastructure of Bruch's membrane. II. Eyes with a tapetum. Arch Ophthalmol 1964;72:388–94.

[9] Park KL. Anatomy of the uvea. In: Yanoff M, Duker JS, editors. Ophthalmology. St. Louis (MO): Mosby; 1999. p. 10:2.1–2.2.

[10] Mafee MF, Peyman GA. Retinal and choroidal detachment: role of MRI and CT. Radiol Clin North Am 1987;25:487–507.

[11] Mafee MF. Magnetic resonance imaging: ocular anatomy and pathology. In: Newton TH, Bilanuik LT, editors. Modern neuroradiology, vol. 4. Radiology of the eye and orbit. New York: Clavadel press/Raven press; 1990. p. 2.1–3.45.

[12] Mafee MF, Goldberg MF, Valvassori GE, et al. Computed tomography in the evaluation of patients with persistent hyperplastic primary vitreous (PHP's). Radiology 1982;145:713–4.

[13] Anand R. Serous detachment of the neural retina. In: Yanoff M, Duker JS, editors. Ophthalmology. St. Louis (MO): Mosby; 1999. p. 8:40.1–40.6.

[14] Mafee MF, Peyman GA. Choroidal detachment and ocular hypotony: CT evaluation. Radiology 1984;153:697–703.

[15] Peyman GA, Mafee MF, Schulman JA. Computed tomography in choroidal detachment. Ophthalmology 1984;92:156–62.

[16] Mafee MF, Linder B, Peyman GA, et al. Choroidal hematoma and effusion: evaluation with MR imaging. Radiology 1988;168:781–6.

[17] Capper SA, Leopold IH. Mechanism of serous choroidal detachment. Arch Ophthalmol 1956; 55:101–13.

[18] Siegelman J, Jakobiec FA, Eisner G, editors. Retinal diseases: pathogenesis, laser therapy and surgery. Boston: Little, Brown; 1984. p. 1–66.

[19] Kapusta MA, Lopez PF. Choroidal hemorrhage. In: Yanoff M, Duker JS, editors. Ophthalmology. St. Louis (MO): Mosby; 1999. p. 41.1–8:41.4.

[20] Goldstein DA, Tessler HH. Episcleritis, scleritis and other scleral disorders. In: Yanoff M, Duker JS, editors. Ophthalmology. St. Louis (MO): Mosby; 1999. p. 5:13.1–13.9.

[21] Chaques VJ, Lam S, Tessler HH, et al. Computed tomography and magnetic resonance imaging in the diagnosis of posterior scleritis. Ann Ophthalmol 1993;25:89–94.

[22] Forster DJ. Basic principles: general approach to the uveitis patient and treatment strategies. In: Yanoff M, Duker JS, editors. Ophthalmology. St. Louis (MO): Mosby; 1999. p. 10:3.1–3.6.

[23] Marx JL. Endophthalmitis. In: Yanoff M, Duker JS, editors. Ophthalmology. St. Louis (MO): Mosby; 1999. p. 10:21.1–21.6.

[24] Yan X, Edward DP, Mafee MF. Ocular calcification: radiologic-pathologic correlation and literature review. International Journal of Neuroradiology 1998;4:81–96.

[25] Zeffer HJ. Calcification and ossification in ocular tissue. Am J Ophthalmol 1983;101:1724–7.

[26] Bullock JD, Campbell RJ, Waller RR. Calcification in retinoblastoma. Invest Ophthalmol Vis Sci 1976;11:252–5.

[27] Mafee MF, Peyman GA, McKusick MA. Malignant uveal melanoma and similar lesions studied by computed tomography. Radiology 1985;156: 403–8.

[28] Mafee MF, Peyman GA, Grisolano JE, et al. Malignant uveal melanoma and simulating le-

sions: MR imaging evaluation. Radiology 1986; 160:773–80.

[29] Mafee MF, Peyman GA, Peace JH, et al. MRI in the evaluation and differentiation of uveal melanoma. Ophthalmology 1987;94:341–8.

[30] Mafee MF. Uveal melanoma, choroidal hemangioma, and simulating lesions. Radiol Clin North Am 1998;36:1083–99.

[31] Mafee MF, Goldberg MF, Greenwald MJ, et al. Retinoblastoma and simulating lesion: role of CT and MR Imaging. Radiol Clin North Am 1987; 25:667–81.

[32] Mafee MF, Goldberg MF, Cohen SB, et al. Magnetic resonance imaging of leukokoric eyes and use of in vitro proton magnetic resonance spectroscopy of retinoblastoma. Ophthalmology 1989;96:965–76.

[33] Kaufman LM, Mafee MF, Song CD. Retinoblastoma and simulating lesions: role of CT, MR imaging and use of Gd-DTPA contrast enhancement. Radiol Clin North Am 1998;36:1101–17.

[34] Chavez M, Mafee MF, Castillo B, et al. Medulloepithelioma of the optic nerve. J Pediatr Ophthalmol Strabismus 2004;41:48–52.

[35] Enochs SW, Petherick P, Bogdanova A, et al. Paramagnetic metal scavenging by melanin: MR imaging. Radiology 1997;204:417–23.

[36] Mafee MF, Ainbinder DJ, Hidayat AA, et al. Magnetic resonance imaging and computed tomography in the evaluation of choroidal hemangioma. International Journal of Neuroradiology 1995;1:67–77.

[37] Mafee MF, Atlas SW, Galetta SL. Eye, orbit, and visual system. In: Atlas SW, editor. Imaging of the brain and spine. 3rd edition. Philadelphia: Lippincott Williams & Wilkins; 2002. p. 1433–524.

[38] Mafee MF, Miller MT, Tan W, et al. Dynamic computed tomography and its application to ophthalmology. Radiol Clin North Am 1987; 25:715–31.

RADIOLOGIC
CLINICS
OF NORTH AMERICA

Radiol Clin N Am 44 (2006) 159–164

Index

Note: Page numbers of article titles are in **boldface** type.

0033-8389/06/$ – see front matter © 2005 Elsevier Inc. All rights reserved.
radiologic.theclinics.com

doi:10.1016/S0033-8389(05)00165-X

Changing Your Address?

Make sure your subscription changes too! When you notify us of your new address, you can help make our job easier by including an exact copy of your Clinics label number with your old address (see illustration below.) This number identifies you to our computer system and will speed the processing of your address change. Please be sure this label number accompanies your old address and your corrected address—you can send an old Clinics label with your number on it or just copy it exactly and send it to the address listed below.

We appreciate your help in our attempt to give you continuous coverage. Thank you.

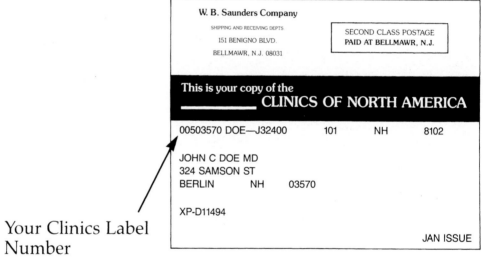

Your Clinics Label Number
Copy it exactly or send your label
along with your address to:
W.B. Saunders Company, Customer Service
Orlando, FL 32887-4800
Call Toll Free 1-800-654-2452

Please allow four to six weeks for delivery of new subscriptions and for processing address changes.